Fight Against Dementia and Alzheimer's Disease: A Patient Survival

A Guide Based On Medical Research

Allen Huff, BS, DC
Self Published E-book

Legal / Medical Disclaimer:

The medical information on this book is provided as an information resource only, and is not to be used or relied on for any diagnostic or treatment purposes. This information is a summary of medical articles and does not create any patient-physician relationship, and should not be used as a substitute for professional diagnosis and treatment.

Please consult your health care provider before making any health care decisions or for guidance about a specific medical condition. Allen Huff expressly disclaims responsibility, and shall have no liability, for any damages, loss, injury, or liability whatsoever suffered as a result of your reliance on the information contained in this book.

The content is not intended to be a substitute for professional medical advice, diagnosis, or treatment. Always seek the advice of a physician or other qualified health provider with any questions you may have regarding a medical condition. Never disregard professional medical advice or delay in seeking it because of something you have read here.

Allen Huff does not endorse specifically any test, treatment, or procedure mentioned on the book.

Dedication:

A continued thanks to my:

El Elyon
Wife Monica
Daughter Olivia
My Best Friend Matt
My Parents Stewart and Jean

Table of Contents:

Copper: ↑ 97

Diabetes: ↑ 106

Exercise: ↓ 115

Fish: ↓ 119

Fish Oil (Omega 3 &DHA): ↓ 125

Free Radicals: ↑ 133

Fruit: ↓ 138

Ginger: ↓ 145

Gingko Biloba: ↓ 148

Glutamate: ↑ 154

Glutathione: ↓ 157

Glyphosate / Round up: ↑ 162

Iron: ↑ 166

Lewy Bodies: ↑ 171

Lipids: ↑ 174

Magnesium: ↓ 179

Medications: ↑ 183

Mercury: ↑ 188

Music: ↓ 193

NSAIDS: ↕ 199

Obesity: ↑ 203

Polyphenols: ↓ 212

Selenium: ↓ 218

Statin: ↕ 223

Foreword:

Boy have times changed! When I was a young boy, we would be pretty keen about what you'd say to your grandparents or even the elderly at large. They were sharp, astute, and keen. From my grandfather playing golf till he was 94, riding his bicycle a few miles a week in his late eighties to my grandmother who was overly serious about bridge and could answer almost all of Alex Trebek's questions in Jeopardy. Was my memory tainted about the elderly?

After having countless conversations with patients over the years, I found out my memories are not as tainted as I had thought. Most of us have memories of people over 70 who were "with it", "sharp", "present". I remember my grandfather taking apart a radio on his workbench when he was over 75 years of age, mumbling about how they didn't make things like they used to.

Over the last 30 years, things have changed dramatically. It can be very tough when I find patients struggling for words, drop a conversation mid dialogue, can't seem to remember important portions of their case history. I once was surprised by a client who forgot he had a double spiral fracture of his left femur and I wondered, HOW!. This year I had a client forget they had a bout with cancer until the third visit!

Just because something has become common place doesn't mean it is normal. When I grew up, the statistics on all sorts of diseases were far less than today. From cancer to autism, you can check any study you want and all of the numbers have gone nothing but up, decade after decade.

"It's in the genes", as a common answer patients whip out when something is wrong. There is _some_ truth here. There are things we can't control when we are adults: our height, our eye color, our skin color, and so on. However, there are dozens of things we **can** control. The below will be an example of what we can do even though we're bound by our DNA.

Our DNA is much like a farm field. Well that farm may be fixed by location and access to water, but we can choose what kind of seed to plant, how to take care of it, whether to fertilize it, whether to prevent weed growth and insects from attacking it, how and when we plant & harvest, and many other attributes associated with taking care of that seed we put in our fixed ground that we own.

We cannot change is the ground we have. We are not allowed to sell or trade but we can work the land differently to produce a different bushel yield of whichever crop our soil is best in adequate for. Our body is much like that field and while we cannot change our DNA; however, our DNA is responsive to what we eat, drink, rest, sleep, stresses and a host of factors we can change. More importantly what we do not put in our bodies can be immensely helpful.

It would make sense to any layperson that anyone who would eat chips, candy bars, soda, high carb high processed food, premade food would produce one type of body compared to a person who never ate any of those and ate fruits, vegetables, nuts, beans, meat raise off the land and eat locally grown foods.

Now it is simple to type this metaphor but we have to fight our nature. I can have a desire to eat sweets, speed when I drive, and a dozen other things that make me "feel" great. But alas, I get in trouble. So I have to put away my desires and behave. But seriously, if we learn to control our desires, we can be healthier. No patient has said: "I never knew that!", but so many didn't know where to start or what to do. So, the following chapters are opportunities to help your body fight back.

The purpose of this book is straight forward: reduce or stop a few things that are **increasing** your statistics of getting dementia and Alzheimer's Disease. Start incorporating some subjects/topics that can help your body **reduce** your current and future statistics. The author would think that it would be great to do this BEFORE you have symptoms. That's it.

Book Format:

The Short Story:
For the nuts & bolts person

Here is just what you need, the subject and the short version that was chosen to help you or a loved one with Alzheimer's and dementia.

The Details:
For the detail orientated person, professional, geek or information hound I have added a section where cited references list more information. Included were some of my favorite commentary but wished to respect the copyright so if you need a few more that a couple of comments, please check out the original article.

From my experience, most patients just want the basics with the ability to back up the ideas, hence the format I choose.

Icons for quick browsing:

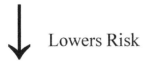 Lowers Risk

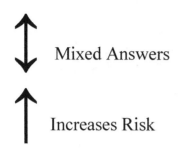 Mixed Answers

Increases Risk

Introduction:

Dementia Defined: a group of symptoms affecting memory, thinking, social relationships, personality changes, inability to distinguish reality from fantasy, impaired reasoning, and onset of interference with normal activities of daily living.

Alzheimer's Disease Defined: a continued progression of dementia where the brain degenerates such that many to most memories are altered or absent, language skills show advanced decline, behaviors to even loved ones can be rude, mean and downright uncalled for. At first, recent memories are altered and as the disease progressed the patient can easily forget a spouse of 40 years or their very own children.

Current Alzheimer's disease medications and management strategies may offer temporary relief or some improvement but today no clear singular answer / cure is available.

Brief statistics about dementia and Alzheimer's:

According to:
http://www.who.int/features/factfiles/dementia/en/
- Worldwide is currently estimated at 47.5 million
- Projected to increase to 75.6 million by 2030.
- Dementia is estimated to more than triple by 2050.
- 58% live in low- and middle-income countries, and this proportion is projected to rise to 71% by 2050.
- The total number of new cases of dementia each year worldwide is nearly 7.7 million, implying 1 new case every 4 seconds.

Other recent statistics:
- About 1 in 8 people age 65 and over have dementia.
- Women are more likely to have it than men.
- Alzheimer's was first discovered in 1906 by Dr. Alois Alzheimer.

Activities: ↓

Games, Puzzles, Video Games, Exercise

The Short Story:
Defined: Physical or mental activities which a person can do to stimulate their brain to prevent or slow the effects of dementia.

Summary: Yes exercise helps, yes puzzles reduce the onset of dementia up to 2.5 years, and yes even non-action video games from the grandparents help!

Lightning facts:
- Physical inactivity **increases risk** factors for dementia. [1.]
- Brain stimulating activity helps keep the cognitive reserve. [1.]
- **Aerobic** activity would slow brain loss the most.
- Healthy **lifestyles** can enhance memory of individuals <u>even with</u> cognitive decline. [2.]
- "...**aerobic** physical fitness program can **partially** serve as a non-medication alternative for maintaining and improving these functions in older adults; however, leisure activities should also be considered." [3.]
- "...training healthy older adults **with non-action video games will** enhance some cognitive abilities but not others." [4.]
- "The largest benefits seem to be provided by **exergames** which combine game play with significant physical exercise." [5.]

- "For **some** individuals, participation in cognitive activities pertinent to game playing **may** help **prevent** AD by preserving brain structures and cognitive functions vulnerable to AD pathophysiology." [6.]
- **Behavior-Based Ergonomic Therapy comprehensive nonpharmacological intervention reduced falls by 32.5%.** [7.]
- "**Crossword puzzle** participation at baseline **delayed onset** of accelerated memory decline by 2.54 years." [8.]

The Details:
According to:
1. Cognitive Reserve and the Prevention of Dementia: the Role of Physical and Cognitive Activities. Curr Psychiatry Rep. 2016 Sep;18(9):85. Cheng ST. doi: 10.1007/s11920-016-0721-2. PMID: 27481112 PMCID: PMC4969323 DOI: 10.1007/s11920-016-0721-2

"The article discusses the two most significant modifiable risk factors for dementia, namely, physical inactivity and lack of stimulating cognitive activity, and their effects on developing cognitive reserve."

"In addition, physical activity, particularly aerobic exercise, is associated with less age-related gray and white matter loss and with less neurotoxic factors. On the other hand, cognitive training studies suggest that training for executive functions (e.g., working memory) improves prefrontal network efficiency, which provides support to brain functioning in the face of cognitive decline."

"While physical activity preserves neuronal structural integrity and brain volume (hardware), cognitive activity strengthens the functioning and plasticity of neural circuits (software), thus supporting cognitive reserve in different ways."

According to:
2. The Effects of Cognitive Training for Elderly: Results from My Mind Project. Rejuvenation Res. 2016 Apr 8. [Epub ahead of print] Giuli C, Papa R, Lattanzio F, et al. PMID: 26952713 DOI: 10.1089/rej.2015.1791

"The aim of this study was to investigate the effects of a nonpharmacological intervention consisting of comprehensive cognitive training in elderly people having one of three different cognitive statuses."

"In the three groups, immediately after the end of the intervention, we observed a significant effect on some cognitive and noncognitive outcomes in the EGs."

"The role of healthy lifestyle programs, such as the use of comprehensive interventions, has been shown to be efficient for enhancing memory and other abilities in aged individuals with and without cognitive decline."

According to:
3. The influence of physical exercise and leisure activity on neuropsychological functioning in older adults. Age (Dordr). 2015 Aug;37(4):9815. Antunes HK, Santos-Galduroz RF, De Aquino Lemos V, et al. doi: 10.1007/s11357-015-9815-8. Epub 2015 Jul 14. PMID: 26169946 PMCID: PMC4501327 DOI: 10.1007/s11357-015-9815-8

"It has been suggested that leisure activity and physical exercise can be a protective factor for neuropsychological functions and are associated with a reduced risk of dementia."

"The data suggest that physical exercise improves neuropsychological functioning, although leisure activities may also improve this functioning. Thus, an aerobic physical fitness program can partially serve as a non-medication alternative for maintaining and improving these functions in older adults; however, leisure activities should also be considered."

According to:
4. Brain training with non-action video games enhances aspects of cognition in older adults: a randomized controlled trial. Ballesteros S, Prieto A, Mayas J, et al. Front Aging Neurosci. 2014 Oct 14;6:277. doi: 10.3389/fnagi.2014.00277. eCollection 2014. PMID: 25352805 PMCID: PMC4196565

Corrigendum: Brain training with non-action video games enhances aspects of cognition in older adults: a randomized controlled trial. [Front Aging Neurosci. 2015]

"This randomized controlled study investigated the effects of 20 1-h non-action video game training sessions with games selected from a commercially available package (Lumosity) on a series of age-declined cognitive functions and subjective wellbeing."

"Overall, the current results support the idea that training healthy older adults with non-action video games will enhance some cognitive abilities but not others."

According to:
5. [The effects of video games on cognitive aging]. Maillot P, Perrot A, Hartley A., et al. Geriatr Psychol Neuropsychiatr Vieil. 2012 Mar;10(1):83-94. PMID: 22414403 DOI: 10.1684/pnv.2012.0317

"Advancing age is associated with cognitive decline, which, however, remains a very heterogeneous phenomenon."

"This review of the literature aims to establish a precise inventory of the relations between the various types of video games and cognitive aging, including both sedentary video games (i.e., classics as well as brain training) and active video games (i.e., exergames)."

"The largest benefits seem to be provided by exergames which combine game play with significant physical exercise."

According to:
6. Participation in cognitively-stimulating activities is associated with brain structure and cognitive function in preclinical Alzheimer's disease. Brain Imaging Behav. 2015 Dec;9(4):729-36. Schultz SA1,2, Larson J1,2, Oh J1,2, et al. PMID: 25358750 PMCID: PMC4417099 [Available on 2016-12-01] DOI: 10.1007/s11682-014-9329-5

"This study tested the hypothesis that frequent participation in cognitively-stimulating activities, specifically those related to playing games and puzzles, is beneficial to brain health and cognition among middle-aged adults at increased risk for Alzheimer's disease (AD)."

"Similarly, Cognitive Activity Scale (CAS)-Games scores were positively associated with scores on the Immediate Memory, Verbal Learning & Memory, and Speed & Flexibility domains."

"For some individuals, participation in cognitive activities pertinent to game playing may help prevent AD by preserving brain structures and cognitive functions vulnerable to AD pathophysiology."

According to:
7. Individualized behavior management program for Alzheimer's/dementia residents using behavior-based ergonomic therapies. Bharwani G1, Parikh PJ, Lawhorne LW, et al. Am J Alzheimers Dis Other Demen. 2012 May;27(3):188-95. PMID: 22517891 DOI: 10.1177/1533317512443869 Epub 2012 Apr 19.

"We develop a comprehensive nonpharmacological intervention, the Behavior-Based Ergonomic Therapy (BBET), which consists of multiple therapies. This low-cost, 24/7 program uses learning, personality, and behavioral profiles and cognitive function of each resident to develop a set of individualized therapies."

"The quantitative and qualitative benefits of the BBET were evaluated at the dementia care unit in a not-for-profit continuing care retirement community in west central Ohio. The 6-month pilot study reduced falls by 32.5% and markedly reduced agitation through increased resident engagement."

According to:
8. Association of crossword puzzle participation with memory decline in persons who develop dementia. Pillai JA, Hall CB, Dickson DW, et al. J Int Neuropsychol Soc. 2011 Nov;17(6):1006-13 PMID: 22040899 PMCID: PMC3885259 DOI: 10.1017/S1355617711001111

"Participation in cognitively stimulating leisure activities such as crossword puzzles may delay onset of the memory decline in the preclinical stages of dementia, possibly via its effect on improving cognitive reserve."

"Crossword puzzle participation at baseline delayed onset of accelerated memory decline by 2.54 years. Inclusion of education or participation in other cognitively stimulating activities did not significantly add to the fit of the model beyond the effect of puzzles."

Advanced Glycation End Products: ↑

The Short Story:
Defined: Proteins or fats that become bound to sugar in high heat. They advance aging and in the development or worsening of many degenerative diseases, such as diabetes, atherosclerosis, kidney failure, and Alzheimer's disease to mention a few.

Summary: Horrible! Stay away from sugar combined with high heat. It byproduct will help destroy DNA, or in geek speak it erodes the telomeres, thus shortening your health and longevity with quality of life.

Lightning facts:
- **Accelerated** of AGEs is Alzheimer's Disease, where AGEs can be detected in amyloid plaques and neurofibrillary tangles. [1.]
- "AGE modification may explain many of the **neuropathological** and biochemical features of AD such as extensive protein cross-linking, **inflammation, oxidative** stress and neuronal cell death." [1.]
- Application of α-lipoic acid **decreased** AGE accumulations. [2.]

- If you want less AGE's consider less of: "**Meat** was always the food with the largest amount of AGEs. Other foods with significant AGEs included **fish, cheese**, vegetables, and vegetable oil." [3.]
- **"This finding is congruent with the epidemiology that has long pointed to only three substantial factors that alter risk of dementia other than age: head injury, anti-inflammatory drugs, and diabetes."** [5.]
- "It is clear that AGEs modification triggers the **abnormal deposition and accumulation** of the modified proteins, which in turn sustain the local **oxidative stress** and **inflammatory** response, eventually **leading** to the pathological and clinical aspects of **neurodegenerative** diseases." [6.]

Tip: Stay away from anything heated that has high meat, fish or cheese combined with sugar. A few examples might be meat lovers pizza, bbq ribs, fish sticks, bacon, …. These would have combined AGE potentials that can cause you unnecessary risk.

The Details:
According to:
1. Advanced glycation end products as biomarkers and gerontotoxins - A basis to explore methylglyoxal-lowering agents for Alzheimer's disease? Krautwald M, Münch G. Exp Gerontol. 2010 Oct;45(10):744-51. doi: 10.1016/j.exger.2010.03.001. Epub 2010 Mar 6. PMID: 20211718

"Alzheimer's disease (AD) is the most common dementing disorder of late life. Although there might be various different triggering events in the early stages of the disease, they seem to converge on a few characteristic final pathways in the late stages, characterized by inflammation and neurodegeneration."

"Accumulation of AGEs is a normal feature of aging, but is accelerated in AD, where AGEs can be detected in amyloid plaques and neurofibrillary tangles. AGE modification may explain many of the neuropathological and biochemical features of AD such as extensive protein cross-linking, inflammation, oxidative stress and neuronal cell death."

According to:
2. Advanced glycation end products are mitogenic signals and trigger cell cycle reentry of neurons in Alzheimer's disease brain. Kuhla A, Ludwig SC, Kuhla B, et al. Neurobiol Aging. 2015 Feb;36(2):753-61. Epub 2014 Oct 13. PMID: 25448604 DOI: 10.1016/j.neurobiolaging.2014.09.025

"Neurons that reenter the cell cycle die rather than divide, a phenomenon that is associated with neurodegeneration in Alzheimer's disease (AD)."

"Because microglia and astroglia proliferate in the vicinity of amyloid plaques, it is likely that plaque components or factors secreted from plaque-activated glia induce neuronal mitogenic signaling."

"Advanced glycation end products (AGEs), protein-bound oxidation products of sugar, might be one of those mitogenic compounds."

"In addition, reduction of oxidative stress by application of α-lipoic acid decreased AGE accumulations, and this decrease was accompanied by a reduction in cell cycle reentry and a more euploid neuronal genome."

According to:
3. Observational and ecological studies of dietary advanced glycation end products in national diets and Alzheimer's disease incidence and prevalence.
Perrone L, Grant WB.   J Alzheimers Dis. 2015;45(3):965-79. doi: 10.3233/JAD-140720. PMID: 25633677 DOI: 10.3233/JAD-140720

"Considerable evidence indicates that diet is an important risk-modifying factor for Alzheimer's disease (AD). Evidence is also mounting that dietary advanced glycation end products (AGEs) are important risk factors for AD."

"Meat was always the food with the largest amount of AGEs. Other foods with significant AGEs included fish, cheese, vegetables, and vegetable oil."

"By using two different models to extrapolate dietary AGE intake in the WHICAP 1992 and 1999 cohort studies, we showed that reduced dietary AGE significantly correlates with reduced AD incidence."

According to:
4. The Possible Mechanism of Advanced Glycation End Products (AGEs) for Alzheimer's Disease. Ko SY, Ko HA, Chu KH, et al. PLoS One. 2015 Nov 20;10(11):e0143345. eCollection 2015. PMID: 26587989 PMCID: PMC4654523 DOI: 10.1371/journal.pone.0143345

"Glyceraldhyde-derived AGEs has been identified as a major source of neurotoxicity in Alzheimer's disease (AD)."

"Our findings suggest that AGEs increase reactive oxygen species (ROS) production, which stimulates downstream pathways related to APP processing, Aβ production, Sirt1, and GRP78, resulting in the up-regulation of cell death related pathway. This in-turn enhances neuronal cell death, which leads to the development of AD."

According to:
5. Advanced glycation end products, dementia, and diabetes. Simon Lovestonea,1 and Ulf Smithb
Proc Natl Acad Sci U S A. 2014 Apr 1; 111(13): 4743–4744. Published online 2014 Mar 25. doi: 10.1073/pnas.1402277111 PMCID: PMC3977311

"The formation and aggregation of Amyloid beta (Aβ) and the phosphorylation and aggregation of tau are clearly part of the core pathogenesis."

"This finding is congruent with the epidemiology that has long pointed to only three substantial factors that alter risk of dementia other than age: head injury, anti-inflammatory drugs, and diabetes."

"It is reasonably clear why head injury and anti-inflammatory drugs might affect risk but the relationship between diabetes and dementia has been far less clear. It could be that diabetes simply increases risk of vascular and related damage to the brain as it does to limbs, kidneys, and other organs."

"In both the mice and also in a human cohort, dietary fed methyl-glyoxyl (MG) levels and accompanying advanced glycation end products (AGEs) correlated positively with cognitive deficits or decline and inversely with survival factor sirtuin-1 (SIRT1) levels and other markers of insulin sensitivity."

"...excess of glycotoxins in particular—suppresses SIRT1 with adverse consequences for both systemic insulin sensitivity and AD pathogenic processes, ... Increased tau phosphorylation disrupts binding to microtubules resulting in a translocation from the axon, a loss of microtubule stability and function, and a tendency to increased aggregation (12), all of which are part of the tau-related toxicity of the disease (13)."

"This theory suggests SIRT1 as the link between pathways that induce insulin resistance..."

"Specifically, the finding that a diet rich in glycotoxins increases the β-cleavage of APP, resulting in Aβ generation, and is accompanied by a decrease in SIRT1 does offer sight of a unifying hypothesis that is in line with previous evidence."

According to:
6. Advanced glycation end products and neurodegenerative diseases: mechanisms and perspective. Li J, Liu D, Sun L, Lu Y, et al. J Neurol Sci. 2012 Jun 15;317(1-2):1-5. doi: 10.1016/j.jns.2012.02.018. Epub 2012 Mar 11. PMID: 22410257 DOI: 10.1016/j.jns.2012.02.018

"The age-related neurodegenerative disorders such as Alzheimer's, Parkinson's, and Huntington's diseases are characterized by the abnormal accumulation or aggregation of proteins. Advanced glycation end products (AGEs) are proteins or lipids that become glycated after exposure to sugars."

"These data suggest that AGEs contribute to the development of neurodegenerative diseases. "

"It is clear that AGEs modification triggers the abnormal deposition and accumulation of the modified proteins, which in turn sustain the local oxidative stress and inflammatory response, eventually leading to the pathological and clinical aspects of neurodegenerative diseases."

According to:
7. The role of advanced glycation end products in various types of neurodegenerative disease: a therapeutic approach. Salahuddin P, Rabbani G, Khan RH. Cell Mol Biol Lett. 2014 Sep;19(3):407-37. Epub 2014 Aug 20. PMID: 25141979 DOI: 10.2478/s11658-014-0205-5

"Protein glycation is initiated by a nucleophilic addition reaction between the free amino group from a protein, lipid or nucleic acid and the carbonyl group of a reducing sugar."

"This review focuses on the pathway of AGE formation, the synthesis of different types of AGE, and the molecular mechanisms by which glycation causes various types of neurodegenerative disease."

"Additionally, the review covers several defense enzymes and proteins in the human body that are important anti-glycating systems acting to prevent the development of neurodegenerative diseases."

Age: ↑

The Short Story:
Defined: Day by day, we each get older. The total U.S. population that ages until we die is 100%.

Summary: It isn't that we age, it is how fast we age. Some people look way younger, some much other than they "should" at a particular age. Take control now and make a difference on each day of the rest of your life and how fast you will age.

Lightning facts:
- **Delaying** retirement **decreases** the risk of dementia. [1.]

- Older people traditionally do **not** like to cook, **decreasing** the quality and frequency of macronutrients (good food) thus **increasing** their **risk** of **earlier** dementia. [2.]

- "Advanced age by itself **failed** to be associated with **decisional incapacity** in this sample." [4.]

- "The incidence of dementia **increases exponentially** with age, and is all too frequent in the oldest old ($\geq$ 90 years of age), the fastest growing age group in many countries." [6.]

- "However, brain pathology and cognitive decline **are not inevitable, even at extremely old age** (den Dunnen et al., 2008)." [6.]

- "There are indications, however, for better cognitive performance and delayed cognitive decline, supporting a link between **female hormone deficiency** and cognitive aging." [7.]
- "Among the 93 identified risk factors, **seven** major modifiable ones should be considered: low **education, sedentary** lifestyle, midlife **obesity**, midlife **smoking, hypertension, diabetes**, and midlife **depression**." [8.] [WOW]
- "Three other important modifiable risk factors should also be added to this list: midlife **hypercholesterolemia**, late life atrial **fibrillation**, and **chronic kidney** disease." [8.]

The Details:
According to:
1. Older age at retirement is associated with decreased risk of dementia. Dufouil C, Pereira E, Chêne G, et al. Eur J Epidemiol. 2014 May;29(5):353-61. Epub 2014 May 4. PMID: 24791704 DOI: 10.1007/s10654-014-9906-3

"To test the hypothesis that age at retirement is associated with dementia risk among self-employed workers in France, we linked health and pension databases of self-employed workers and we extracted data of those who were still alive and retired as of December 31st 2010."

"We show strong evidence of a significant decrease in the risk of developing dementia associated with older age at retirement, in line with the "use it or lose it" hypothesis."

According to:
2. Nutritional strategies to optimise cognitive function in the aging brain. Wahl D1, Cogger VC, Solon-Biet SM, et al. Ageing Res Rev. 2016 Nov;31:80-92. Epub 2016 Jun 26. PMID: 27355990 PMCID: PMC5035589 [Available on 2017-11-01] DOI: 10.1016/j.arr.2016.06.006

"Old age is the greatest risk factor for most neurodegenerative diseases."

"CR (calorie restriction) influences brain aging in many animal models and recent findings suggest that dietary interventions can influence brain health and dementia in older humans."

"One of the primary purposes of this review is to explore the notion that macronutrients may have a more translational potential than CR and IF in humans, and therefore there is a pressing need to use GF to study the impact of diet on brain aging. Furthermore, given the growing recognition of the role of aging biology in dementia, such studies might provide a new approach for dietary interventions for optimizing brain health and preventing dementia in older people.

According to:
3. Dopamine Receptor Genes Modulate Associative Memory in Old Age. Papenberg G, Becker N, Ferencz B, et al. J Cogn Neurosci. 2016 Sep 20:1-9. [Epub ahead of print] PMID: 27647283 DOI: 10.1162/jocn_a_01048

"Previous research shows that associative memory declines more than item memory in aging. Although the underlying mechanisms of this selective impairment remain poorly understood, animal and human data suggest that dopaminergic modulation may be particularly relevant for associative binding."

"Taken together, our results suggest that DA (Dopamine receptor genes) may be particularly important for associative memory, whereas (Alzheimer's Disease) AD-related genetic variations may influence overall episodic memory in older adults without dementia.

According to:
4. Advanced age and decisional capacity: The effect of age on the ability to make health care decisions. Boettger S, Bergman M, Jenewein J, et al. Arch Gerontol Geriatr. 2016 Sep-Oct;66:211-7. Epub 2016 Jun 17. PMID: 27371804 DOI: 10.1016/j.archger.2016.06.011

"Out of more than 2500 consecutive psychiatric consultations performed by the Consultation-Liaison service at Bellevue Hospital Center in New York City, 266 completed decisional capacity assessments were identified and analyzed with respect to the indications for referral and the impact of age and other sociodemographic, medical and psychiatric variables on decisional capacity."

"Advanced age by itself failed to be associated with decisional incapacity in this sample. In those ≥65, cognitive disorders remained the main association with such incapacity, versus psychosis, substance use and neurological disorders in younger patients."

According to:
5. Caregiver burden in family carers of people with dementia with Lewy bodies and Alzheimer's disease. Svendsboe E Terum T, Testad I, et al. Int J Geriatr Psychiatry. 2016 Sep;31(9):1075-83. Epub 2016 Jan 14. PMID: 26765199 DOI: 10.1002/gps.4433

"To characterise the differences in caregiver distress between carers of people diagnosed with dementia with Lewy bodies (DLB) and people with Alzheimer's disease (AD), with a view to differentiating and improving support for caregivers."

"This study is a part of two larger Norwegian studies, DemVest (n = 265) and The Norwegian Dementia Register (n = 2220), with data from caregivers and people diagnosed with AD (n = 100) and DLB (n = 86) between 2005 and 2013. The average age was 74.9 years (SD = 7.8)."

"Caregivers to people with AD (20.2%) and 40% of caregivers for people with DLB experienced moderate or high caregiver burden with an increased risk of psychiatric disorders in the early stage of dementia."

According to:
6. Preserved brain metabolic activity at the age of 96 years. Apostolova I, Lange C, Spies L, et al. Int Psychogeriatr. 2016 Sep;28(9):1575-7. Epub 2016 May 10. PMID: 27160670 DOI: 10.1017/S1041610216000673

"Loss of brain tissue becomes notable to cerebral magnetic resonance imaging (MRI) at age 30 years, and progresses more rapidly from mid 60s."

"The incidence of dementia increases exponentially with age, and is all too frequent in the oldest old (≥ 90 years of age), the fastest growing age group in many countries."

"However, brain pathology and cognitive decline are not inevitable, even at extremely old age (den Dunnen et al., 2008)."

According to:
7. Age at menopause and duration of reproductive period in association with dementia and cognitive function: A systematic review and meta-analysis. Georgakis MK, Kalogirou EI, Diamantaras AA, et al. Psychoneuro-endocrinology. 2016 Nov;73:224-243. Epub 2016 Aug 3. PMID: 27543884 DOI: 10.1016/j.psyneuen.2016.08.003

"The preponderance of dementia among postmenopausal women compared with same-age men and the female sex hormones neuroprotective properties support a tentative role of their deficiency in the dementia pathogenesis."

"Age at menopause (13 studies; 19,449 participants) and reproductive period (4 studies; 9916 participants) in the highest categories were not associated with odds of dementia (effect size [ES]: 0.97 [0.78-1.21]) and Alzheimer's disease (ES: 1.06 [0.71-1.58])."

"There are indications, however, for better cognitive performance and delayed cognitive decline, supporting a link between female hormone deficiency and cognitive aging."

According to:
8. Is It Possible to Delay or Prevent Age-Related
Cognitive Decline? Michel JP. Korean J Fam Med. 2016
Sep;37(5):263-6. Epub 2016 Sep 21. PMID: 27688858
DOI: 10.4082/kjfm.2016.37.5.263

"After two decades of lack of success in dementia drug
discovery and development, and knowing that worldwide,
currently 36 million patients have been diagnosed with
Alzheimer's disease, a number that will double by 2030
and triple by 2050, the World Health Organization and the
Alzheimer's Disease International declared that prevention
of cognitive decline was a 'public health priority.'"

"Among the 93 identified risk factors, seven major
modifiable ones should be considered: low education,
sedentary lifestyle, midlife obesity, midlife smoking,
hypertension, diabetes, and midlife depression."

"Three other important modifiable risk factors should also
be added to this list: midlife hypercholesterolemia, late life
atrial fibrillation, and chronic kidney disease."

Aluminum: ↑

The Short Story:

Defined: Aluminium, a.k.a. aluminum, is a chemical element with symbol Al and atomic number 13.

Summary: Aluminum damages the brain, memory, and messes with our gut functions. Find it and take it out of anything you can.

Email me for an image of where Aluminum is hiding in the products we use or consume. My email is book@nucca.info.

Lightning facts:

- "Even when Al and Pb can reach and **accumulate** in **almost every organ** in the human body, the central **nervous system** is a particular target of the **deleterious effects** of both metals." [1]
- Aluminum **damages** the brain. [2]
- Aluminum + Copper = brain **inflammation**. [2]
- Aluminum affects brain cells called microglia and astrocytes.
- "… **long-term** persistence of aluminum adjuvants in humans results in cognitive **dysfunction**, affecting **visual** and **verbal** memory, as well as executive functions such as attention, **working memory** and planning." [2]
- Two types of aluminum have **high** absorption from the **gut** and passage into the brain. [2]

- Diet affects dementia: [3.]
  - **Decrease** dementia by:
    - 16% with Unsaturated Fatty Acids
    - 13% with antioxidants,
    - 28% with vitamin B
    - 31% with Mediterranean diet
  - **Increase** dementia by:
    - 224% with aluminum
    - 43% with smoking
    - 152% with low Vitamin D
- Results showed that individuals **chronically** exposed to Al were **71% more** likely to develop AD. [4.]
- "In other neurodegenerative disorders, Cu, zinc, aluminum and manganese are involved." [5.]
- "Al is considered as a well-established neurotoxin and have a link between the exposure and development of neurodegenerative diseases, including Amyotrophic Lateral Sclerosis (ALS), Alzheimer's disease (AD), dementia, Gulf war syndrome and Parkinsonism." [6.]
- From a review of **34 studies**: "The findings of the present meta-analyses demonstrate that **aluminum** levels are **significantly** elevated in brain, serum, and CSF of patients with AD." [8.]
- "… (1) aluminum's absorption rates, allowing the impression that aluminum is safe to ingest and as an **additive in food and drinking water treatment**, (2) aluminum's **slow** progressive uptake into the **brain** over a **long** prodromal phase, and (3) aluminum's similarity to iron, in terms of ionic size, allows aluminum to use iron-evolved mechanisms to enter the highly-active, iron-dependent cells responsible for **memory** processing." [10.]

- "The physical properties of aluminum and ferric iron ions are similar, allowing aluminum to use mechanisms evolved for iron to enter vulnerable neurons involved in AD progression, accumulate in those neurons, and cause neurofibrillary damage." [11].

The Details:
According to:
1. Aluminium and lead: molecular mechanisms of brain toxicity. Verstraeten SV, Aimo L, Oteiza PI. Arch Toxicol. 2008 Nov;82(11):789-802. doi: 10.1007/s00204-008-0345-3. Epub 2008 Jul 31. PMID: 18668223

"The fact that aluminium (Al) and lead (Pb) are both toxic metals to living organisms, including human beings, was discovered a long time ago. Even when Al and Pb can reach and accumulate in almost every organ in the human body, the central nervous system is a particular target of the deleterious effects of both metals."

"Select human population can be at risk of Al neurotoxicity, and Al is proposed to be involved in the etiology of neurodegenerative diseases. Pb is a widespread environmental hazard, and the neurotoxic effects of Pb are a major public health concern."

According to:
2. Aluminum Induced Immunoexcitotoxicity in Neuro-developmental and Neurodegenerative Disorders Current Inorganic Chemistry. Russell L. Blaylock, MD 2012, Vol. 2, No. 1

"Aluminum and aluminofluoride compounds activate the brain's innate immune system (microglia) releasing neurotoxic concentrations of excitotoxins [glutamate / aspartate] and pro-inflammatory cytokines, chemokines and immune mediators. This damages the brain."

"Metal ions, including aluminum drive crosstalk between cytokine (immune) receptors and glutamate (excitatory) receptors, called immunoexcitotoxicity."

"Aluminum "is a major neurotoxin and disrupter of neurological function. Aluminum in combination with copper additively increases brain inflammation,""

"When humans are exposed to aluminum via parenteral fluids and/or vaccines, it is "completely absorbed and distributed throughout the body."

"Microglia and astrocytes are sites of preferential aluminum accumulation and toxic action. When activated, microglia can secrete pro-inflammatory cytokines and excitotoxins."

"… long-term persistence of aluminum adjuvants in humans results in cognitive dysfunction, affecting visual and verbal memory, as well as executive functions such as attention, working memory and planning."

"Two forms of aluminum are of special concern: aluminum-L-glutamate and nanoscaled aluminum, both of which have high absorption from the gut and passage into the brain, as well as higher toxicity profiles than aluminum alone."

According to:
3. Dietary Patterns and Risk of Dementia: a Systematic Review and Meta-Analysis of Cohort Studies. Cao L, Tan L, Wang HF, et al. Mol Neurobiol. 2015 Nov 9. PMID: 26553347 DOI: 10.1007/s12035-015-9516-4

"Dietary patterns and some dietary components have been linked with dementia. We therefore performed a meta-analysis of available studies to determine whether there is an association between diet and risk of dementia."

"Some food intake was related with decrease of dementia, such as unsaturated fatty acids (RR: 0.84, 95 % CI: [0.74-0.95], $P = 0.006$), antioxidants (RR: 0.87, 95 % CI: [0.77-0.98], $P = 0.026$), vitamin B (RR: 0.72, 95 % CI: [0.54-0.96], $P = 0.026$), and the Mediterranean diet (MeDi) (RR: 0.69, 95 % CI: [0.57-0.84], $P < 0.001$)."

"Some material intakes were related with increase of dementia, such as aluminum (RR: 2.24, 95 % CI: [1.49-3.37], $P < 0.001$), smoking (RR: 1.43, 95 % CI: [1.15-1.77], $P = 0.001$), and low levels of vitamin D (RR: 1.52, 95 % CI: [1.17-1.98], $P = 0.002$)."

According to:
4. Chronic exposure to aluminum and risk of Alzheimer's disease: A meta-analysis. Wang Z, Wei X, Yang J, et al. Neurosci Lett. 2016 Jan 1;610:200-6. Epub 2015 Nov 27. PMID: 26592479 DOI: 10.1016/j.neulet.2015.11.014

"A meta-analysis was performed to investigate whether chronic exposure to aluminum (Al) is associated with increased risk of Alzheimer's disease (AD). Eight cohort and case-control studies (with a total of 10567 individuals) that met inclusion criteria for the meta-analysis were selected after a thorough literature review of PubMed, Web of Knowledge, Elsevier ScienceDirect and Springer databases up to June, 2015."

"Results showed that individuals chronically exposed to Al were 71% more likely to develop AD (OR: 1.71, 95% confidence interval (CI), 1.35-2.18). The finding suggests that chronic Al exposure is associated with increased risk of AD."

According to:
5. Brain biometals and Alzheimer's disease - boon or bane? Prakash A, Dhaliwal GK, Kumar P, et al. Int J Neurosci. 2016 Apr 25:1-10. PMID: 27044501 DOI: 10.3109/00207454.2016.1174118

"Alzheimer's disease (AD) is the most common form of dementia."

"Biometals play an important role in the normal body functioning but AD may be mediated or triggered by disproportion of metal ions leading to changes in critical biological systems and initiating a cascade of events finally leading to neurodegeneration and cell death."

"The link is multifactorial, and although the source of the shift in oxidative homeostasis is still unclear, current evidence points to changes in the balance of redox transition metals, especially iron, copper (Cu) and other trace metals. Their levels in the brain are found to be elevated in AD. In other neurodegenerative disorders, Cu, zinc, aluminum and manganese are involved."

According to:
6. Multifaceted effects of aluminium in neurodegenerative diseases: A review. Biomed Pharmacother. 2016 Jul 29;83:746-754. Maya S, Prakash T, Madhu KD, et al. PMID: 27479193 DOI: 10.1016/j.biopha.2016.07.035

"However, the evidence suggests that the Al can potentiate oxidative stress and inflammatory events and finally leads to cell death."

"Al is considered as a well-established neurotoxin and have a link between the exposure and development of neurodegenerative diseases, including Amyotrophic Lateral Sclerosis (ALS), Alzheimer's disease (AD), dementia, Gulf war syndrome and Parkinsonism."

"This review summarizes Al induced events likewise oxidative stress, cell mediated toxicity, apoptosis, inflammatory events in the brain, glutamate toxicity, effects on calcium homeostasis, gene expression and Al induced Neurofibrillary tangle (NFT) formation."

According to:

7. What is the risk of aluminium as a neurotoxin? Exley C. Expert Rev Neurother. 2014 Jun;14(6):589-91. Epub 2014 Apr 30. PMID: 24779346 DOI: 10.1586/14737175.2014.915745

"Aluminium is neurotoxic. Its free ion, Al(3+) (aq), is highly biologically reactive and uniquely equipped to do damage to essential cellular (neuronal) biochemistry."

"Aluminium is present in the human brain and it accumulates with age. The most recent research demonstrates that a significant proportion of individuals older than 70 years of age have a potentially pathological accumulation of aluminium somewhere in their brain."

According to:
8. Aluminum Levels in Brain, Serum, and Cerebrospinal Fluid are Higher in Alzheimer's Disease Cases than in Controls: A Series of Meta-Analyses. Virk SA, Eslick GD. J Alzheimers Dis. 2015;47(3):629-38. PMID: 26401698 DOI: 10.3233/JAD-150193

"Overall, 34 studies involving 1,208 participants and 613 AD cases met the criteria for inclusion. Aluminum was measured in brain tissue in 20 studies (n=386), serum in 12 studies (n=698), and CSF in 4 studies (n=124)."

"Compared to control subjects, AD sufferers had significantly higher levels of brain (SMD 0.88; 95% CI, 0.25-1.51), serum (SMD 0.28; 95% CI, 0.03-0.54), and CSF (SMD 0.48; 95% CI, 0.03-0.93) aluminum."

"The findings of the present meta-analyses demonstrate that aluminum levels are significantly elevated in brain, serum, and CSF of patients with AD. These findings suggest that elevated aluminum levels, particularly in serum, may serve as an early marker of AD and/or play a role in the development of the disease."

According to:
9. Brain biometals and Alzheimer's disease - boon or bane? Prakash A, Dhaliwal GK, Kumar 2,et al. Int J Neurosci. 2016 Apr 25:1-10. PMID: 27044501 DOI: 10.3109/00207454.2016.1174118

"It is attributed to a variety of pathological conditions that share similar critical processes, such as oxidative stress, proteinaceous aggregations, mitochondrial dysfunctions and energy failure. There is increasing evidence suggesting that metal homeostasis is dysregulated in the pathology of AD."

"The link is multifactorial, and although the source of the shift in oxidative homeostasis is still unclear, current evidence points to changes in the balance of redox transition metals, especially iron, copper (Cu) and other trace metals."

According to:
10. Chronic aluminum intake causes Alzheimer's disease: applying Sir Austin Bradford Hill's causality criteria. Walton JR1. J Alzheimers Dis. 2014;40(4):765-838. PMID: 24577474 DOI: 10.3233/JAD-132204

"Industrialized societies produce many convenience foods with aluminum additives that enhance various food properties and use alum (aluminum sulfate or aluminum potassium sulfate) in water treatment to enable delivery of large volumes of drinking water to millions of urban consumers."

"Mechanisms that underlie the risk of low concentrations of aluminum relate to (1) aluminum's absorption rates, allowing the impression that aluminum is safe to ingest and as an additive in food and drinking water treatment, (2) aluminum's slow progressive uptake into the brain over a long prodromal phase, and (3) aluminum's similarity to iron, in terms of ionic size, allows aluminum to use iron-evolved mechanisms to enter the highly-active, iron-dependent cells responsible for memory processing."

"Aluminum particularly accumulates in these iron-dependent cells to toxic levels, dysregulating iron homeostasis and causing microtubule depletion, eventually producing changes that result in disconnection of neuronal afferents and efferents, loss of function and regional atrophy consistent with MRI findings in AD brains."

According to:

11. Aluminum involvement in the progression of Alzheimer's disease. Walton JR1. J Alzheimers Dis. 2013;35(1):7-43. PMID: 23380995 DOI: 10.3233/JAD-121909

"Chronic aluminum neurotoxicity best matches this profile. Many humans routinely ingest aluminum salts as additives contained in processed foods and alum-treated drinking water."

"The physical properties of aluminum and ferric iron ions are similar, allowing aluminum to use mechanisms evolved for iron to enter vulnerable neurons involved in AD progression, accumulate in those neurons, and cause neurofibrillary damage."

"This review describes evidence for aluminum involvement in AD neuropathology and the clinical progression of sporadic AD."

APOE E4
Gene ↕

The Short Story:
Defined: APOE (Apolipoprotein E) is a class of proteins on your 19th chromosome.

Summary: Depending on which set of genes (E2, E3, & E4) you received from your mother and father (determined by genetic testing) it can increase or decrease your risk of getting Alzheimer's Disease.

Lightning facts:
- "The association of increased allele frequency of APOE4 with Alzheimer's disease has been reproduced in several dozen laboratories around the world." [1]
- 8 times the risk of Alzheimer's Disease if you have one Ɛ4 gene and are recently depressed. [2]
- 10 times the risk of Alzheimer's Disease if you have one Ɛ4 gene and are clinical-verified depression. [2]
- 7 times the risk of Alzheimer's Disease if you have one Ɛ4 gene and are reporting sleep disturbance. [2]

The Details:
According to:
http://alzdiscovery.org/cognitive-vitality/blog/what-apoe-means-for-your-health

---

48

In order to break down complex material I have referenced two images to help us.

The below chart was included because of its simplicity and information. In each column are the outcomes you can have based on each gene your parent gave you.

Genotype	E2/E2	E2/E3	E2/E4	E3/E3	E3/E4	E4/E4
Disease Risk	40% less likely	40% less likely	2.6 times more likely	Average risk	3.2 times more likely	14.9 times more likely

The next image will show the complex relationship of the APOE E4 gene and risks.

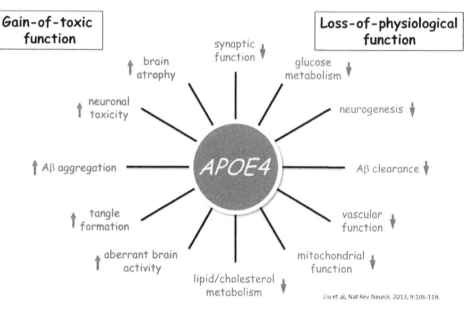

Liu, et al, Nat Rev Neurol, 2013; 9:106-118.

According to:

1. APOE is a major susceptibility gene for Alzheimer's disease. Roses AD, Saunders AM. Curr Opin Biotechnol. 1994 Dec;5(6):663-7. PMID: 7765750

"The initial report on APOE as a susceptibility gene for late-onset Alzheimer's disease was presented a little more than two years ago."

"The association of increased allele frequency of APOE4 with Alzheimer's disease has been reproduced in several dozen laboratories around the world."

"The role of apoE as a metabolic co-factor in neuronal metabolism presents new possibilities for neuronal mechanisms of maintenance and response to stress."

According to:
2. Associations between depression, sleep disturbance, and apolipoprotein E in the development of Alzheimer's disease: dementia. Burke SL, Maramaldi P, Cadet T, et al. Int Psychogeriatr. 2016 Sep;28(9):1409-24. doi: 10.1017/S1041610216000405.

"Within the US, AD is the most common form of dementia in the elderly, affecting 1 in 10 people over the age of 65."

"Sleep disturbance has been called a "public health epidemic" and, like depression, is a prodromal symptom of AD but may also contribute to the risk of developing AD."

"It was hypothesized that sleep disturbance, depression, and the apolipoprotein E (APOE) genotype increase the likelihood of AD."

"The hazard of developing AD was eight times higher for those with recent depression and the Ɛ4 homozygote (HR = 8.15 [3.70-17.95]). Among Ɛ4 carriers with clinician-verified depression, the hazard was ten times that of the reference group (HR = 10.11 [4.43-23.09]). The hazard for Ɛ4 carriers reporting sleep disturbance was almost 7 times greater than the reference group (HR = 6.79 [2.38-19.37])."

Aspirin: ↑

The Short Story:
Defined: A white, crystalline compound derived from salicylic acid. A.K.A. acetylsalicylic acid.

Summary: Taking a daily aspirin is **not** some small thing or to be taken lightly. It **doesn't** help Alzheimer's Disease, it can increase hemorrhaging in your brain, the safety coating could **increase** the speed and risk of AD.

Lightning facts:
- Buffered aspirin has 50 mg Al per serving. [1.]
- Aspirin is **only** recommended to prevent the **second** and **not** the first heart attack or stroke. [1.]
- The coating that **protects** the stomach from ulcers is from the aluminum that has been **strongly linked** to Alzheimer's Disease. [1.]
- Aspirin, steroids, traditional NSAIDs and selective COX-2 inhibitors do not help cognitive decline BUT aspirin increases more bleeding. [2.]
- An interesting side note of **NSAIDs** increased blood pressure and trend towards **higher** death rates, even worse in selective COX-2 inhibitors. [2.]
- In a small study: "...aspirin use was associated with **greater** prospective cognitive decline on select measures, potentially reflecting its common use for vascular disease prophylaxis." [3.]
- A study showed **no** evidence to support a potential protective effect of NSAIDs against dementia. [4.]

52

- In a small study, **aspirin** use in AD might pose an **increased** risk of intracerebral hemorrhage (ICH), whereas it has no effect on cognition. [5.]

The Details:
According to:
1. Use of Aspirin for Primary Prevention of Heart Attack and Stroke. 12/16/16.
http://www.fda.gov/Drugs/ResourcesForYou/Consumers/ucm390574.htm

"The FDA has reviewed the available data and **does not** believe the evidence supports the general use of aspirin for primary prevention of a heart attack or stroke. In fact, there are serious risks associated with the use of aspirin, including increased risk of bleeding in the stomach and brain, in situations where the benefit of aspirin for primary prevention has not been established."

"The available evidence **supports** the use of aspirin for preventing **another** heart attack or stroke in patients who have **already** had a heart attack or stroke, or have other evidence of coronary artery disease, such as angina or a history of a coronary bypass operation or coronary angioplasty."

"The most common side effect from regular aspirin usage is upper abdominal pain from gastric irritation."

"Enteric coasted aspirin is recommended to deal with this. 8 The coating supposedly prevents inflammation of the stomach lining but contains aluminum, around 50 mg. per pill 9 Aluminum has been strongly linked with the development of Alzheimers Disease.10"

According to:
2. Aspirin, steroidal and non-steroidal anti-inflammatory drugs for the treatment of Alzheimer's disease. Jaturapatporn D, Isaac MG, McCleery J, et al. Cochrane Database Syst Rev. 2012 Feb 15;(2):CD006378. doi: 10.1002/14651858.CD006378.pub2.

"To review the efficacy and side effects of aspirin, steroidal and non-steroidal anti-inflammatory drugs (NSAIDs) in the treatment of AD, compared to placebo."

"Our search identified 604 potentially relevant studies. Of these, 14 studies (15 interventions) were RCTs and met our inclusion criteria. The numbers of participants were 352, 138 and 1745 for aspirin, steroid and NSAIDs groups, respectively."

"There was no significant improvement in cognitive decline for aspirin, steroid, traditional NSAIDs and selective COX-2 inhibitors. Compared to controls, patients receiving aspirin experienced more bleeding while patients receiving steroid experienced more hyperglycaemia, abnormal lab results and face edema."

"Patients receiving NSAIDs experienced nausea, vomiting, elevated creatinine, elevated LFT and hypertension. A trend towards higher death rates was observed among patients treated with NSAIDS compared with placebo and this was somewhat higher for selective COX-2 inhibitors than for traditional NSAIDs."

According to:
3. Nonsteroidal anti-inflammatory drugs, aspirin, and cognitive function in the Baltimore longitudinal study of aging. Waldstein SR, Wendell CR, Seliger SL, et al. J Am Geriatr Soc. 2010 Jan;58(1):38-43. PMID: 20122039 PMCID: PMC2832849 DOI: 10.1111/j.1532-5415.2009.02618.x

"To examine the relations between the use of nonaspirin, nonsteroidal anti-inflammatory drugs (NSAIDs) and aspirin and age-related change in multiple domains of cognitive function in community-dwelling individuals without dementia."

"Longitudinal, with measures obtained on one to 18 occasions over up to 45 years."

"In contrast, aspirin use was associated with greater prospective cognitive decline on select measures, potentially reflecting its common use for vascular disease prophylaxis. Effect sizes were small, calling into question clinical significance, although overall public health significance may be meaningful."

According to:
4. NSAID Use and Incident Cognitive Impairment in a Population-based Cohort. Wichmann MA, Cruickshanks KJ, Carlsson CM, et al.
Alzheimer Dis Assoc Disord. 2016 Apr-Jun;30(2):105-12. PMID: 26079710 PMCID: PMC4670291 [Available on 2017-04-01] DOI: 10.1097/WAD.0000000000000098

"Nonsteroidal anti-inflammatory drugs (NSAIDs) may prevent dementia, but previous studies have yielded conflicting results."

"Participants using aspirin at baseline but not 5 years prior were more likely to develop cognitive impairment (adjusted hazard ratio=1.77; 95% confidence interval=1.11, 2.82; model 2), with nonsignificant associations for longer term use."

"Nonaspirin NSAID use was not associated with incident cognitive impairment or mild cognitive impairment/dementia odds. These results provided no evidence to support a potential protective effect of NSAIDs against dementia."

According to:
5. Aspirin in Alzheimer's disease: increased risk of intracerebral hemorrhage: cause for concern? Thoonsen H, Richard E, Bentham P, Gray R, et al. Stroke. 2010 Nov;41(11):2690-2. doi: 10.1161/STROKEAHA.109.576975. Epub 2010 Oct 7.

"Systematic review and comparison of the occurrence of events over time between the aspirin and control group in each trial using Cox regression analysis."

"Although the number of cases in both trials is small, our findings suggest that aspirin use in AD might pose an increased risk of ICH, whereas it has no effect on cognition. If there is an unequivocal cardiovascular indication for aspirin, it should not be withheld in AD patients."

Broccoli: ↓

The Short Story:
Defined: A cultivated vegetable from the cruciferous family.

Summary: Eating broccoli helps put an important but rare compound in your body to **fight plaques** that increase dementia and Alzheimer's Disease.

Lightning facts:

- A compound in broccoli called **sulforaphane** (SFN) is able to **protect** the brain from Alzheimer-like lesions. [1.]

- Sulforaphane **significantly reduced** damage to specific areas of AD brains. [2.]

- Sulforaphane makes neurobehavioral deficits **better** from "**cholinergic** nerve damage" [3.]; see my chapter titled medications for pharmacy causes of AD.

- Therefore, sulforaphane appears to be a **promising** compound with neuroprotective properties that may play an important role in **preventing** neurodegeneration." [4.]

- "While the exact mechanism of interaction of SFN in AD has not yet been ascertained, our results suggest that SFN can **aid in cognitive impairment** and may **protect** the brain from amyloidogenic damages." [5.]

The Details:
According to:
1. Sulforaphane ameliorates neurobehavioral deficits and protects the brain from amyloid β deposits and peroxidation in mice with Alzheimer-like lesions. Zhang R, Miao QW, Zhu CX, et al. Am J Alzheimers Dis Other Demen. 2015 Mar;30(2):183-91. Epub 2014 Jul 13. PMID: 25024455 DOI: 10.1177/1533317514542645

"Alzheimer's disease (AD) is a common neurodegenerative disease in the elderly individuals and its effective therapies are still unavailable."

"This study was designed to investigate the neuroprotection of sulforaphane (SFN) in AD-lesion mice induced by combined administration of d-galactose and aluminium."

"In conclusion, SFN ameliorates neurobehavioral deficits and protects the brain from Aβ deposits and peroxidation in mice with Alzheimer-like lesions, suggesting SFN is likely a potential phytochemical to be used in AD therapeutics."

According to:
2. Sulforaphane exerts its anti-inflammatory effect against amyloid-β peptide via STAT-1 dephosphorylation and activation of Nrf2/HO-1 cascade in human THP-1 macrophages. An YW, Jhang KA, Woo SY, et al. Neurobiol Aging. 2016 Feb;38:1-10. Epub 2015 Oct 23. PMID: 26827637 DOI: 10.1016/j.neurobiolaging.2015.10.016

"Alzheimer's disease (AD) is the most common neurodegenerative disorder worldwide, accounting for most cases of dementia in elderly individuals, and effective therapies are still lacking."

"The anti-inflammatory effect of sulforaphane on $A\beta1$-42-induced IL-1β production was diminished by small interfering RNA-mediated knockdown of Nrf2 or HO-1."

"Moreover, sulforaphane significantly attenuated the levels of microRNA-146a, which is selectively upregulated in the temporal cortex and hippocampus of AD brains."

"These findings suggest that the phytochemical sulforaphane has a potential application in AD therapeutics."

According to:
3. Neuroprotective effects of sulforaphane on cholinergic neurons in mice with Alzheimer's disease-like lesions. Int J Mol Sci. 2014 Aug 18;15(8):14396-410. Zhang R, Zhang J, Fang L, et al. PMID: 25196440 PMCID: PMC4159858 DOI: 10.3390/ijms150814396

"This study was designed to investigate the neuroprotective effects of sulforaphane (an activator of NF-E2-related factor 2) on mice with AD-like lesions induced by combined administration of aluminum and D-galactose."

"Step-down-type passive avoidance tests showed sulforaphane ameliorated cognitive impairment in AD-like mice."

"In conclusion, sulforaphane ameliorates neurobehavioral deficits by reducing cholinergic neuron loss in the brains of AD-like mice, and the mechanism may be associated with neurogenesis and aluminum load reduction. These findings suggest that phytochemical sulforaphane has potential application in AD therapeutics."

According to:
4. Sulforaphane as a potential protective phytochemical against neurodegenerative diseases. Tarozzi A, Angeloni C, Malaguti M, et al. Oxid Med Cell Longev. 2013;2013:415078. Epub 2013 Jul 25. PMID: 23983898 PMCID: PMC3745957 DOI: 10.1155/2013/415078

"As no drugs are available to prevent the progression of these neurological disorders, intervention strategies using phytochemicals have been proposed as an alternative form of treatment."

"In particular, evidence suggests that sulforaphane beneficial effects could be mainly ascribed to its peculiar ability to activate the Nrf2/ARE pathway. Therefore, sulforaphane appears to be a promising compound with neuroprotective properties that may play an important role in preventing neurodegeneration."

According to.:
5. Amelioration of Alzheimer's disease by neuroprotective effect of sulforaphane in animal model. Kim HV, Kim HY, Ehrlich HY, et al. Amyloid. 2013 Mar;20(1):7-12. Epub 2012 Dec 19. PMID: 23253046 DOI: 10.3109/13506129.2012.751367

"Pathophysiological evidences of AD have indicated that aggregation of Aβ is one of the principal causes of neuronal dysfunction, largely by way of inducing oxidative stresses such as free radical formation."

"We hypothesized that the known antioxidative attribute of SFN could be harnessed in Alzheimer's treatment."

"While the exact mechanism of interaction of SFN in AD has not yet been ascertained, our results suggest that SFN can aid in cognitive impairment and may protect the brain from amyloidogenic damages."

Brussels Sprouts: ↓

The Short Story:
Defined: This is a form of cabbage which help us avoid chronic, excessive inflammation.

Summary: Eating just a few of these can help **fight plaques** from building up in your brain.

Lightning facts:
- Brussel sprouts have ingredients that **protect against DNA-damage**. [1.]
- "Our study shows for the first time that sprout **consumption** leads to **inhibition** of sulfotransferases in humans and to protection against PhIP and **oxidative DNA-damage**." [1.]
- "Brussels sprouts could be **protective** against amyloid beta (Aβ)-induced **neurotoxicity**, possibly due to the antioxidative capacity of its major constituent, **kaempferol**." [2.]

The Details:
According to:
1. Consumption of Brussels sprouts protects peripheral human lymphocytes against 2-amino-1-methyl-6-phenylimidazo[4,5-b]pyridine (PhIP) and oxidative DNA-damage: results of a controlled human intervention trial.

Hoelzl C, Glatt H, Meinl W, et al. Mol Nutr Food Res. 2008 Mar;52(3):330-41. doi: 10.1002/mnfr.200700406. PMID: 18293303 [PubMed - indexed for MEDLINE]

"To find out if the cancer protective effects of Brussels sprouts seen in epidemiological studies are due to protection against DNA-damage, an intervention trial was conducted in which the impact of vegetable consumption on DNA-stability was monitored in lymphocytes with the comet assay."

"After consumption of the sprouts (300 g/p/d, n = 8), a reduction of DNA-migration (97%) induced by the heterocyclic aromatic amine 2-amino-1-methyl-6-phenyl-imidazo-[4,5-b]pyridine (PhIP) was observed whereas no effect was seen with 3-amino-1-methyl-5H-pyrido[4,3-b]-indole (Trp-P-2)."

"Our study shows for the first time that sprout consumption leads to inhibition of sulfotransferases in humans and to protection against PhIP and oxidative DNA-damage."

According to:
2. Effects of brussels sprouts and their phytochemical components on oxidative stress-induced neuronal damages in PC12 cells and ICR mice. Kim JK, Shin EC, Kim CR, et al. J Med Food. 2013 Nov;16(11):1057-61. doi: 10.1089/jmf.2012.0280. Epub 2013 Oct 31. PMID: 24175656 DOI: 10.1089/jmf.2012.0280

———

"In this study, the protective effects of Brussels sprouts extract and its major constituents against oxidative stress-induced damages were investigated in rat pheochromocytoma cells and Institute of Cancer Research mice."

"Taken together, the results suggest that Brussels sprouts could be protective against amyloid beta (Aβ)-induced neurotoxicity, possibly due to the antioxidative capacity of its major constituent, kaempferol."

Carbohydrates: ↑

The Short Story:
Defined: A molecule of food that is easily converted into sugars.

Summary: The **less** carbs you eat starting now, the better your brain will function as you age.

Lightning facts:

- "Older people who **load** up their **plates** with **carbohydrates** have nearly **four times the risk** of developing mild cognitive impairment, a new study finds." [1.]

- "Those whose diets were **highest in fat** (nuts, healthy oils) were **42% less** likely to get cognitive impairment, while those who had the **highest intake of protein** (chicken, meat, fish) had a **reduced risk of 21%**." [1.]

- "…contrary to normal cells, **most malignant cells depend on steady glucose** availability in the blood for their energy…" [2.]

- "… chronic ingestion of CHO-rich Western diet meals, can **directly promote tumor cell** proliferation via the insulin/IGF1 signaling pathway." [2.]

- "In conclusion, the dietary recommendations for the **prevention and management** of AD are a high consumption of fish, vegetables, and low glycemic index fruits; a moderate amount of meat and dairy products; and **a lower amount of carbohydrates and refined sugar.**" [3.]
- If you are diabetic at midlife (A1C>6.5-11) you have a 32% higher risk of dementia-related death than those with levels less than 5.1. [4.]

The Details:
According to:
1. Relative intake of macronutrients impacts risk of mild cognitive impairment or dementia. Roberts RO, Roberts LA, Geda YE, et al. J Alzheimers Dis. 2012;32(2):329-39. doi: 10.3233/JAD-2012-120862. PMID: 22810099 PMCID: PMC3494735 DOI: 10.3233/JAD-2012-120862

Also see: http://www.j-alz.com/press/2012/20121016.html a Mayo Clinic Study 16-October-2012 - Eating Lots of Carbs, Sugar May Raise Risk of Cognitive Impairment, Mayo Clinic Study Finds

"Older people who load up their plates with carbohydrates have nearly four times the risk of developing mild cognitive impairment, a new study finds."

"Sugars also played a role in the development of MCI, which is often a precursor to Alzheimer's disease"

"Compared with people who rank in the bottom 20% for carbohydrate consumption, those in the highest 20% had a 3.68 times greater risk of MCI, the study found."

"Those whose diets were highest in fat (nuts, healthy oils) were 42% less likely to get cognitive impairment, while those who had the highest intake of protein (chicken, meat, fish) had a reduced risk of 21%."

According to:
2. Is there a role for carbohydrate restriction in the treatment and prevention of cancer? Klement RJ, Kämmerer U. Nutr Metab (Lond). 2011 Oct 26;8:75. doi: 10.1186/1743-7075-8-75. PMID: 22029671 PMCID: PMC3267662 DOI: 10.1186/1743-7075-8-75

"Over the last years, evidence has accumulated suggesting that by systematically reducing the amount of dietary carbohydrates (CHOs) one could suppress, or at least delay, the emergence of cancer, and that proliferation of already existing tumor cells could be slowed down."

"CHOs or glucose, to which more complex carbohydrates are ultimately digested, can have direct and indirect effects on tumor cell proliferation: first, contrary to normal cells, most malignant cells depend on steady glucose availability in the blood for their energy and biomass generating demands and are not able to metabolize significant amounts of fatty acids or ketone bodies due to mitochondrial dysfunction."

"Second, high insulin and insulin-like growth factor (IGF)-1 levels resulting from chronic ingestion of CHO-rich Western diet meals, can directly promote tumor cell proliferation via the insulin/IGF1 signaling pathway."

"In addition, many cancer patients exhibit an altered glucose metabolism characterized by insulin resistance and may profit from an increased protein and fat intake."

According to:
3. [Prevention of Alzheimer's Disease and Nutrients]. Otsuka M. Brain Nerve. 2016 Jul;68(7):809-17. doi: 10.11477/mf.1416200513. [Article in Japanese] PMID: 27395465 DOI: 10.11477/mf.1416200513

"The dietary recommendations for the prevention and management of Alzheimer's disease (AD), are the Mediterranean diet and the Japanese-style diet, both of which contain well-balanced nutrients from fish and vegetables."

"Another nutritional topic with regard to dementia and diet is the association of type-2 diabetes and hyperinsulinemia with AD. Expression array data of the brain tissue of AD patients in the Hisayama study strongly suggests a disturbance in insulin signaling in the AD brain."

"In conclusion, the dietary recommendations for the prevention and management of AD are a high consumption of fish, vegetables, and low glycemic index fruits; a moderate amount of meat and dairy products; and a lower amount of carbohydrates and refined sugar."

According to:
4. Association Between Random Measured Glucose Levels in Middle and Old Age and Risk of Dementia-Related Death. Rosness TA, Engedal K, Bjertness E, et al. J Am Geriatr Soc. 2016 Jan;64(1):156-61. PMID: 26782866 DOI: 10.1111/jgs.13870

"To investigate the association between random measured glucose levels in middle and old age and dementia-related death."

"Individuals without diabetes mellitus at midlife with glucose levels between 6.5 and 11.0 mmol/L had a significantly greater risk of dementia-related death than those with levels less than 5.1 mmol/L (hazard ratio=1.32, 95% confidence interval=1.04-1.67) in a fully adjusted model."

"High random glucose levels measured in middle-aged but not older age persons without known diabetes mellitus were associated with greater risk of dementia-related death up to four decades later."

Caloric Restriction: ↓

<u>The Short Story:</u>
Defined: Reduction of caloric intake via a planned diet to prevent the loss of essential nutrients.

Summary: Caloric restriction via diet helps improve patients even with mild cognitive impairment but unintentional weight loss (usually skipping meals / crappy eating as we age) will increase our risk up to 24%!

Lightning facts:
- A small study found a **significant increase** (20%) of **verbal** memory scores after caloric restriction. [1.]
- "**Obesity** in midlife is a **risk** factor for dementia." [2.]
- "Intentional weight **loss** through **diet** was associated with cognitive improvement in patients with MCI." [2.] (With diet = good or less MCI)
- A Mayo Clinic study suggested: "These findings suggest that increasing weight loss per decade from midlife to late life is a marker for MCI and may help identify persons at increased risk for MCI." [3.]
  - "A weight loss of 5 kg per **decade** corresponds to a 24% increase in risk of MCI" [3.]
  - Hence, **unintentional weight loss** has been associated with an **increased** risk of dementia.

70

o This is when people skip meals, eat quick soups, drink "meal in a can"… that can unintentionally result in slow weight loss. Good intent horrible result due to malnutrition.

- "Strategies for prevention of AD through nonpharmacological treatments are associated with lifestyle interventions such as **exercise**, mental **challenges**, and **socialization** as well as **caloric restriction** and a healthy **diet**." [4.]

- **Increasing** brain-derived neurotrophic factors (BDNF) by **caloric restriction** and **physical** activities has been shown to help **improve** brain function and **long-term memory**. [5.]

The Details:

According to:

1. Caloric restriction improves memory in elderly humans. A. V. Witte,a M. Fobker,b R. Gellner,c S., et al. Proc Natl Acad Sci U S A. 2009 Jan 27; 106(4): 1255–1260. doi: 10.1073/pnas.0808587106 PMCID: PMC2633586

"Animal studies suggest that diets low in calories and rich in unsaturated fatty acids (UFA) are beneficial for cognitive function in age."

"We found a significant increase in verbal memory scores after caloric restriction (mean increase 20%; $P < 0.001$), which was correlated with decreases in fasting plasma levels of insulin and high sensitive C-reactive protein, most pronounced in subjects with best adherence to the diet (all r values < -0.8; all P values <0.05)."

"To our knowledge, the current results provide first experimental evidence in humans that caloric restriction improves memory in the elderly."

"Our findings further point to increased insulin sensitivity and reduced inflammatory activity as mediating mechanisms, leading to higher synaptic plasticity and stimulation of neuroprotective pathways in the brain."

According to:
2. Cognitive Effects of Intentional Weight Loss in Elderly Obese Individuals With Mild Cognitive Impairment. Horie NC, Serrao VT, Simon SS, et tal. J Clin Endocrinol Metab. 2016 Mar;101(3):1104-12. doi: 10.1210/jc.2015-2315. Epub 2015 Dec 29. PMID: 26713821 DOI: 10.1210/jc.2015-2315

"Obesity in midlife is a risk factor for dementia, but it is unknown if caloric restriction-induced weight loss could prevent cognitive decline and therefore dementia in elderly patients with cognitive impairment."

"Eighty obese patients with MCI, aged 60 or older (68.1 ± 4.9 y, body mass index [BMI] 35.5 ± 4.4 kg/m(2), 83.7% women, 26.3% APOE allele ε4 carriers)."

"Intentional weight loss through diet was associated with cognitive improvement in patients with MCI."

According to:

3. Decline in Weight and Incident Mild Cognitive Impairment: Mayo Clinic Study of Aging. JAMA Neurol. Alhurani RE, Vassilaki M, Aakre JA, et al. 2016 Apr;73(4):439-46. doi: 10.1001/jamaneurol.2015.4756. PMID: 26831542 PMCID: PMC4828256

"Because mild cognitive impairment (MCI) is a prodromal stage for dementia, we sought to evaluate whether changes in weight and body mass index (BMI) may predict incident MCI."

"Over a mean follow-up of 4.4 years, 524 of 1895 cognitively normal participants developed incident MCI (50.3% were men; mean age, 78.5 years)."

"A greater decline in weight per decade was associated with an increased risk of incident MCI (hazard ratio [HR], 1.04 [95% CI, 1.02-1.06]; P < .001) after adjusting for sex, education, and apolipoprotein E (APOE) ε4 allele."

"A weight loss of 5 kg per decade corresponds to a 24% increase in risk of MCI (HR, 1.24)."

"These findings suggest that increasing weight loss per decade from midlife to late life is a marker for MCI and may help identify persons at increased risk for MCI."

According to:
4. Therapies for Prevention and Treatment of Alzheimer's Disease. Mendiola-Precoma J, Berumen LC, Padilla K,et al. Biomed Res Int. 2016;2016:2589276. Epub 2016 Jul 28. doi: 10.1155/2016/2589276. PMID: 27547756 PMCID: PMC4980501

"Alzheimer's disease (AD) is the most common cause of dementia associated with a progressive neurodegenerative disorder, with a prevalence of 44 million people throughout the world in 2015, and this figure is estimated to double by 2050."

"Obesity is a major risk factor for AD, because it induces adipokine dysregulation, which consists of the release of the proinflammatory adipokines and decreased anti-inflammatory adipokines, among other processes."

"Strategies for prevention of AD through nonpharmacological treatments are associated with lifestyle interventions such as exercise, mental challenges, and socialization as well as caloric restriction and a healthy diet."

According to:
5. Serum brain-derived neurotrophic factor and the risk for dementia: the Framingham Heart Study. Weinstein G, Beiser AS, Choi SH, et al. JAMA Neurol. 2014 Jan;71(1):55-61. PMID: 24276217 PMCID: PMC4056186 DOI: 10.1001/jamaneurol.2013.4781

"In animal studies, brain-derived neurotrophic factor (BDNF) has been shown to impact neuronal survival and function and improve synaptic plasticity and long-term memory."

"Circulating BDNF levels increase with physical activity and caloric restriction, thus BDNF may mediate some of the observed associations between lifestyle and the risk for dementia."

"Framingham Study original and offspring participants were followed up from 1992 and 1998, respectively, for up to 10 years."

"Compared with the bottom quintile, BDNF levels in the top quintile were associated with less than half the risk for dementia and AD (hazard ratio, 0.49; 95% CI, 0.28-0.85; $P = .01$; and hazard ratio, 0.46; 95% CI, 0.24-0.86; $P = .02$, respectively)."

"Higher serum BDNF levels may protect against future occurrence of dementia and AD. Our findings suggest a role for BDNF in the biology and possibly in the prevention of dementia and AD, especially in select subgroups of women and older and more highly educated persons."

Cerebral Blood Flow (Low): ↑

The Short Story:
Defined: How much blood flows through the brain in a minute, usually measured in milliliters. This can represent 15-20% of our cardiac output at any given time.

Summary: Lower flow rates in our brain change the function of specific tissues related to working memory, reasoning, and function. Research suggest we **increase** (fight back against the risk) this by: stop smoking, meditation, breathing exercises or exercise.

Lightning facts:
- "We found **significant** interactions between diagnosis and CBF for language and between diagnosis and parietal CBF for global **cognition** and **executive functioning**." [1]
- Significant associations between **lower** blood flow inside the head and the **functions** / health of that part of the brain, specifically **emotional** processing (prefrontal cortex) and **higher cognitive** functions and particularly to **working memory** (WM) (superior frontal gyri). [2]

The Details:

According to:

1. Lower cerebral blood flow is associated with impairment in multiple cognitive domains in Alzheimer's disease. Leeuwis AE, Benedictus MR, Kuijer JP, et al. Alzheimers Dement. 2016 Sep 27. pii: S1552-5260(16)32893-X. PMID: 27693109 DOI: 10.1016/j.jalz.2016.08.013[Epub ahead of print]

"We examined the association between decreased cerebral blood flow (CBF) and cognitive impairment in Alzheimer's disease (AD), mild cognitive impairment (MCI), and subjective cognitive decline (SCD)."

"We included 161 AD, 95 MCI, and 143 SCD patients from the Amsterdam Dementia Cohort."

"We found significant interactions between diagnosis and CBF for language and between diagnosis and parietal CBF for global cognition and executive functioning."

"Our results suggest that CBF may have potential as a functional marker of disease severity."

According to:

2. Positive affect and regional cerebral blood flow in Alzheimer's disease.Hayashi S, Terada S, Sato S, et al. Psychiatry Res. 2016 Sep 13;256:15-20. PMID: 27640073 DOI: 10.1016/j.pscychresns.2016.09.003 [Epub ahead of print]

"One hundred sixteen consecutive patients with AD were recruited from the outpatient units of the Memory Clinic of Okayama University Hospital."

"After removing the effects of age, sex, duration of education, and cognitive function, positive affect scores showed a significant correlation with regional cerebral blood flow in the left premotor and superior frontal gyri."

"The left premotor and superior frontal area is significantly involved in the pathogenesis of the decrease of positive affect in AD."

According to:
3. Lower cerebral blood flow is associated with faster cognitive decline in Alzheimer's disease. Benedictus MR, Leeuwis AE, Binnewijzend MA, et al. Eur Radiol. 2016 Jun 22. [Epub ahead of print] PMID: 27334014 DOI: 10.1007/s00330-016-4450-z

"To determine whether lower cerebral blood flow (CBF) is associated with faster cognitive decline in patients with Alzheimer's disease (AD)."

"We included 88 patients with dementia due to AD from the Amsterdam Dementia Cohort."

"Lower CBF, in particular in the posterior brain regions, may have value as a prognostic marker for rate of cognitive decline in AD."

Cholesterol (High): ↑

The Short Story:
Defined: Cholesterol is a steroid and as well as a fat / lipid thought to promote narrowing of the arteries.

Summary: Surprising as it is, the cholesterol we **eat nor** the cholesterol we have in our **circulation** have a hill of beans to do with the disease in our brain. But the **breakdown** of the **metabolism** of cholesterol **inside** the brain does have great **significant** risk to developing mild cognitive impairment which leads to Alzheimer's Disease.

Lightning facts:
- Cholesterol **reduces** the function of brain's center ranging from attention to interoception and subjective awareness: pain, hunger, sounds, and responses like fight or flight. [1.]
- Brain cholesterol is **not dependent on diet** nor is it related to the cholesterol our liver makes from carbs and sugar as it **can't** make it through the blood brain barrier. [2.]
- "… a relationship between plasma cholesterol level and neurodegenerative disorders, such as Alzheimer's disease (AD), has often been reported." [2.]

- Levels of HDL and relation to apolipoproteins A-I and B are **not** to be used as markers to predict AD. [3.]

- "The brain has **elaborate regulatory** mechanisms to control cholesterol metabolism that are **distinct** from the mechanisms in **periphery**." [4.]

- "Interestingly, **dysregulation** of the cholesterol metabolism is **strongly** associated with a number of neurodegenerative diseases." [4.]

- Genetic testing for the **APOE rs429358** variation which has a significant influenced the brain network characteristics would be a **useful** screening for AD and MCI. [5.]

- **Too much** cholesterol combined with a **breakdown** of cholesterol metabolism in the brain will **increase** the risk of AD. [6.]

- **Midlife elevated serum cholesterol** levels and **high blood** pressure play a significant role in developing mild cognitive impairment which leads to Alzheimer's Disease. [7.]

- "Brain cholesterol is primarily derived by de novo synthesis and the blood brain barrier **prevents** the uptake of lipoprotein cholesterol from the circulation." [8.]

- If you measure the concentrations of 24(S)-hydroxycholesterol, the exclusive metabolite of CNS cholesterol, you can monitor the level of cholesterol in the brain and make sure it is not diminishing, thus a risk of AD. [8.]

The Details:

According to:

1. Impacts of High Serum Total Cholesterol Level on Brain Functional Connectivity in Non-Demented Elderly. Zhang T, Li H, Zhang J, et al. J Alzheimers Dis. 2015;50(2):455-63. doi: 10.3233/JAD-150810. PMID: 26682694 DOI: 10.3233/JAD-150810

"Epidemiological and clinical studies suggest that high serum cholesterol is a risk factor of dementia."

"Our findings suggest that in non-demented elderly persons, high serum cholesterol is associated with disruption of functional connectivity in the salience network (SN)."

According to:

2. The Role of Brain Cholesterol and its Oxidized Products in Alzheimer's Disease. Giudetti AM, Romano A, Lavecchia AM, et al. Curr Alzheimer Res. 2016;13(2):198-205. PMID: 26391039

"The human brain is the most cholesterol-rich organ harboring 25% of the total cholesterol pool of the whole body. Cholesterol present in the central nervous system (CNS) comes, almost entirely, from the endogenous synthesis, being circulating cholesterol unable to cross the blood-brain barrier (BBB)."

"Within the brain, cholesterol is transported by HDL-like lipoproteins associated to apoE which represents the main apolipoprotein in the CNS."

"Although CNS cholesterol content is largely independent of dietary intake or hepatic synthesis, a relationship between plasma cholesterol level and neurodegenerative disorders, such as Alzheimer's disease (AD), has often been reported."

"Therefore a special attention was dedicated to the study of the main factors controlling cholesterol metabolism in the brain."

According to:
3. Apolipoproteins and HDL cholesterol do not associate with the risk of future dementia and Alzheimer's disease: the National Finnish population study (FINRISK). Tynkkynen J, Hernesniemi JA, Laatikainen T, et al. Age (Dordr). 2016 Sep 23. [Epub ahead of print] PMID: 27663235 DOI: 10.1007/s11357-016-9950-x

"Data on associations of apolipoproteins A-I and B (apo A-I, apo B) and HDL cholesterol (HDL-C) with dementia and Alzheimer's disease (AD) are conflicting."

"We analyzed the results from two Finnish prospective population-based cohort studies in a total of 13,275 subjects aged 25 to 74 years with mainly Caucasian ethnicity. The follow-up time for both cohorts was 10 years."

"Our study does not support the use of these risk markers to predict incident dementia or AD."

According to:
4. MicroRNAs in brain cholesterol metabolism and their implications for Alzheimer's disease. Yoon H, Flores LF, Kim J. Biochim Biophys Acta. 2016 May 4. pii: S1388-1981(16)30116-0. doi: 10.1016/j.bbalip.2016.04.020. PMID: 27155217 DOI: 10.1016/j.bbalip.2016.04.020

"Cholesterol is important for various neuronal functions in the brain. Brain has elaborate regulatory mechanisms to control cholesterol metabolism that are distinct from the mechanisms in periphery."

"Interestingly, dysregulation of the cholesterol metabolism is strongly associated with a number of neurodegenerative diseases."

"Recently, several microRNAs are demonstrated to be involved in regulating cholesterol metabolism in the brain."

According to:
5. Multiple genetic imaging study of the association between cholesterol metabolism and brain functional alterations in individuals with risk factors for Alzheimer's disease. Bai F, Yuan Y, Shi Y, et al. Oncotarget. 2016 Mar 29;7(13):15315-28. PMID: 26985771 PMCID: PMC4941243 DOI: 10.18632/oncotarget.8100.

"Alzheimer's disease (AD) is a clinically and genetically heterogeneous neurodegenerative disease. Genes involved in cholesterol metabolism may play a role in the pathological changes of AD. "

"A cholesterol metabolism pathway gene-based imaging genetics approach was then utilized to investigate disease-related differences between the groups based on genotype-by-aMCI interactions."

"The APOE rs429358 variation significantly influenced the brain network characteristics, affecting the activation of nodes as well as the connectivity of edges in aMCI subjects."

According to:
6. Imbalanced cholesterol metabolism in Alzheimer's disease. Xue-shan Z, Juan P, Qi W, et al. 2016 May 1;456:107-14. doi: 10.1016/j.cca.2016.02.024. Epub 2016 Mar 2. PMID: 26944571 DOI: 10.1016/j.cca.2016.02.024

"Alzheimer's disease (AD) is a complex and multifactorial neurodegenerative disease that is mainly caused by β-amyloid accumulation."

"A large number of studies have shown that elevated cholesterol levels may perform a function in AD pathology, and several cholesterol-related gene polymorphisms are associated with this disease."

"We first, review metabolism and regulation of the cholesterol in the brain. Second, we summarize the literature stating that hypercholesterolemia is one of the risk factors of AD. Third, we discuss the main mechanisms of abnormal cholesterol metabolism that increase the risk of AD. Finally, the relationships between AD and apolipoprotein E, PCSK9, and LRP1 are discussed in this article."

According to:
7. Midlife vascular risk factors and late-life mild cognitive impairment: A population-based study. Kivipelto M, Helkala EL, Hänninen T, et al. Neurology. 2001 Jun 26;56(12):1683-9. PMID: 11425934 [PubMed - indexed for MEDLINE]

"To evaluate the impact of midlife elevated serum cholesterol levels and blood pressure on the subsequent development of mild cognitive impairment (MCI) and to investigate the prevalence of MCI in elderly Finnish population, applying the MCI criteria devised by the Mayo Clinic Alzheimer's Disease Research Center."

"Eighty-two subjects, 6.1% of the population (average age, 72 years) met the criteria for MCI. Midlife elevated serum cholesterol level (> or =6.5 mmol/L) was a significant risk factor for MCI (OR, 1.9; 95% CI, 1.2 to 3.0, adjusted for age and body mass index); the effect of systolic blood pressure approached significance."

According to:
8. Cholesterol: Its Regulation and Role in Central Nervous System Disorders. M Orth, S. Bellosta, et al. Volume 2012 (2012), Article ID 292598, 19 pages http://dx.doi.org/10.1155/2012/292598 103163, 70199 Stuttgart, Germany

"Cholesterol is a major constituent of the human brain, and the brain is the most cholesterol-rich organ."

"Brain cholesterol is primarily derived by de novo synthesis and the blood brain barrier prevents the uptake of lipoprotein cholesterol from the circulation."

"Defects in cholesterol metabolism lead to structural and functional central nervous system diseases such as Smith-Lemli-Opitz syndrome, Niemann-Pick type C disease, and Alzheimer's disease."

"Cholesterol is an important structural component of cellular membranes and myelin and a precursor of oxysterols, steroid hormones, and bile acids."

"Cholesterol is tightly regulated between the major brain cells—neurons and glia, that is, astrocytes, microglia, and oligodendrocytes—and is essential for normal brain development."

"Cholesterol depletion leads to synaptic and dendritic spine degeneration, failed neurotransmission, and decreased synaptic plasticity [7]."

"However, whole CNS cholesterol production can be very elegantly studied by analyzing the concentrations of 24(S)-hydroxycholesterol, the exclusive metabolite of CNS cholesterol."

"From current understanding, CNS cholesterol is an auspicious target for preventing or even treating Alzheimer's disease."

Coconut Oil: ↓

The Short Story:
Defined: The fatty oil obtained from the coconut.

Summary: There has been a lot of hype and articles pressed about coconut oil and helping dementia to Alzheimer's Disease. There are just a handful of articles in all of PubMed and the below two are noting benefits to help dementia and Alzheimer's Disease. That said, and I see no harm in taking it, but it is the OPINION of this author that there many better choices for your money and a proven scientific trusted result.

Lightning facts:
- Treatment with **40 ml/day** of extra virgin coconut oil **did create improvement** in women > men who **specifically** didn't have Type I diabetes for helping their brain function. [1]
- Coconut oil is being reviewed as an energy source for brain tissue. [2]

The Details:
According to:
1. [COCONUT OIL: NON-ALTERNATIVE DRUG TREATMENT AGAINST ALZHEIMER´S DISEASE]. [Article in Spanish; Abstract available in Spanish from the publisher] Hu Yang I, De la Rubia Ortí JE, Selvi Sabater P, et al. Nutr Hosp. 2015 Dec 1;32(6):2822-7. PMID: 26667739 DOI: 10.3305/nh.2015.32.6.9707

87

"As for treatment, there is no definitive cure drug, thus new therapies are needed. In this regard the medium chain triglycerides are a direct source of cellular energy and can be a nonpharmacological alternative to the neuronal death for lack of it, that occurs in Alzheimer patients."

"…40 ml/day of extra virgin coconut oil."

"It was observed in subjects taking the product, a statistically significant increase in test score MECWOLF and therefore an improvement in cognitive status, improving especially women's, those without diabetes mellitus type II, and severe patients."

According to:
2. The role of dietary coconut for the prevention and treatment of Alzheimer's disease: potential mechanisms of action. Fernando WM, Martins IJ, Goozee KG,et al. Br J Nutr. 2015 Jul 14;114(1):1-14. Epub 2015 May 22. PMID: 25997382 DOI: 10.1017/S0007114515001452

"Unlike most other dietary fats that are high in long-chain fatty acids, coconut oil comprises medium-chain fatty acids (MCFA). MCFA are unique in that they are easily absorbed and metabolised by the liver, and can be converted to ketones."

"It is rich in dietary fibre, vitamins and minerals; however, notably, evidence is mounting to support the concept that coconut may be beneficial in the treatment of obesity, dyslipidaemia, elevated LDL, insulin resistance and hypertension - these are the risk factors for CVD and type 2 diabetes, and also for AD."

"The purpose of the present review was to explore the literature related to coconut, outlining the known mechanistic physiology, and to discuss the potential role of coconut supplementation as a therapeutic option in the prevention and management of AD."

Coffee: ↓

The Short Story:
Defined: Alzheimer's disease (AD) is a progressive, degenerative disorder that attacks the brain's nerve cells, or neurons, resulting in loss of memory, thinking and language skills, and behavioral changes.

Summary: Coffee used long-term helps Alzheimer's, is preventative, and reduces risk at up to **3-5 cups a day**. Study after study proves coffee helps.

Lightning facts:
- **Daily** coffee and caffeine intake does **not** need to be **stopped** in elderly people. [1]
- "Lifelong coffee/caffeine consumption has been associated with **prevention** of **cognitive decline**, and **reduced** risk of developing **stroke, Parkinson's disease** and **Alzheimer's disease**." [1]
- Coffee along with folate, vitamin E &C are considered protective factors against AD. [2]
- Coffee could have **beneficial** effects against **dementia** and **Alzheimer's disease**. [3]
- Coffee and caffeine are known to **enhance** short-term **memory** and **cognition**. [4]
- **Long**-term use of coffee may **protect** against **cognitive decline** or **dementia**. [4]
- Drinking **more** coffee lowers your risk of diabetes mellitus, various cancer lines, Parkinsonism, and Alzheimer's disease. [5]

- Drinking of **3-5 cups per day at midlife** has a **decreased** risk of **dementia/AD by about 65%** at late-life. [6.] WOW

Other facts discovered but not ignored:
"An array of evidence showed that **pregnant** women or those with **postmenopausal** problems should **avoid excessive** consumption of coffee because of its <u>interference</u> with **oral contraceptives** or **postmenopausal hormones**." [5.] Read my chapter below on pregnancy for more details.

The Details:
According to:
1. Effects of coffee/caffeine on brain health and disease: What should I tell my patients? Pract Neurol. 2015 Dec 16. pii: practneurol-2015-001162. Nehlig A. doi: 10.1136/practneurol-2015-001162. PMID: 26677204

"Over the last decade, Food Regulation Authorities have concluded that coffee/caffeine consumption is not harmful if consumed at levels of 200 mg in one sitting (around 2½ cups of coffee) or 400 mg daily (around 5 cups of coffee)."

"In addition, caffeine has many positive actions on the brain. It can increase alertness and well-being, help concentration, improve mood and limit depression."

"Lifelong coffee/caffeine consumption has been associated with prevention of cognitive decline, and reduced risk of developing stroke, Parkinson's disease and Alzheimer's disease."

According to:
2. Meta-analysis of modifiable risk factors for Alzheimer's disease. J Neurol Neurosurg Psychiatry. 2015 Dec;86(12):1299-306. Xu W, Tan L, Wang HF doi: 10.1136/jnnp-2015-310548. Epub 2015 Aug 20. PMID: 26294005

"The aim of our present systematic review and meta-analysis was to roundly evaluate the association between AD and its modifiable risk factors."

"16,906 articles were identified of which 323 with 93 factors met the inclusion criteria for meta-analysis. Among factors with relatively strong evidence (pooled population >5000) in our meta-analysis, we found grade I evidence for 4 medical exposures (oestrogen, statin, antihypertensive medications and non-steroidal anti-inflammatory drugs therapy) as well as 4 dietary exposures (folate, vitamin E/C and coffee) as protective factors of AD."

According to:
3. Gas chromatography time-of-flight mass spectrometry (GC-TOF-MS)-based metabolomics for comparison of caffeinated and decaffeinated coffee and its implications for Alzheimer's disease. PLoS One. 2014 Aug 6;9(8):e104621. Chang KL, Ho PC. doi: 10.1371/journal.pone.0104621. eCollection 2014. PMID: 25098597

"Findings from epidemiology, preclinical and clinical studies indicate that consumption of coffee could have beneficial effects against dementia and Alzheimer's disease (AD)."

"Discriminant metabolites identified in this study are biologically relevant and provide valuable insights into therapeutic research of coffee against AD. Our data also hint at possible involvement of gut microbial metabolism to enhance therapeutic potential of coffee components, which represents an interesting area for future research."

According to:
4. Current evidence for the use of coffee and caffeine to prevent age-related cognitive decline and Alzheimer's disease. J Nutr Health Aging. 2014 Apr;18(4):383-92. Carman AJ, Dacks PA, Lane RF, et al. doi: 10.1007/s12603-014-0021-7. PMID: 24676319

"Although nothing has been proven conclusively to protect against cognitive aging, Alzheimer's disease or related dementias, decades of research suggest that specific approaches including the consumption of coffee may be effective."

"While coffee and caffeine are known to enhance short-term memory and cognition, some limited research also suggests that long-term use may protect against cognitive decline or dementia."

According to:
5. Coffee and its consumption: benefits and risks. Crit Rev Food Sci Nutr. 2011 Apr;51(4):363-73. Butt MS, Sultan MT. doi: 10.1080/10408390903586412. PMID: 21432699

"Coffee is the leading worldwide beverage after water and its trade exceeds US $10 billion worldwide."

"Many research investigations, epidemiological studies, and meta-analyses regarding coffee consumption revealed its inverse correlation with that of diabetes mellitus, various cancer lines, Parkinsonism, and Alzheimer's disease."

"Furthermore, caffeine and its metabolites help in proper cognitive functionality. Coffee lipid fraction containing cafestol and kahweol act as a safeguard against some malignant cells by modulating the detoxifying enzymes."

"An array of evidence showed that pregnant women or those with postmenopausal problems should avoid excessive consumption of coffee because of its interference with oral contraceptives or postmenopausal hormones."

According to:
6. Caffeine as a protective factor in dementia and Alzheimer's disease. J Alzheimers Dis. 2010;20 Suppl 1:S167-74. Eskelinen MH, Kivipelto M. doi: 10.3233/JAD-2010-1404. PMID: 20182054

"In the CAIDE study, coffee drinking of 3-5 cups per day at midlife was associated with a decreased risk of dementia/AD by about 65% at late-life. In conclusion, coffee drinking may be associated with a decreased risk of dementia/AD." (Cardiovascular Risk Factors, Aging and Dementia Study)

According to:
7. Caffeine and coffee as therapeutics against Alzheimer's disease. J Alzheimers Dis. 2010;20 Suppl 1:S117-26. Arendash GW, Cao C. doi: 10.3233/JAD-2010-091249. PMID: 20182037

"Epidemiologic studies have increasingly suggested that caffeine/coffee could be an effective therapeutic against Alzheimer's disease (AD)."

"These results indicate a surprising ability of moderate caffeine intake (the human equivalent of 500 mg caffeine or 5 cups of coffee per day) to protect against or treat AD in a mouse model for the disease and a therapeutic potential for caffeine against AD in humans."

Copper: ↑

The Short Story:
Defined: A reddish metallic element, used in electricity and cooking. This element is essential to life.

Summary: Copper significantly accelerates lipid peroxidation (free radical damage) and is therefore a factor in **accelerating** mild cognitive impairment (MCI) = hurts brain tissue.

Lightning facts:
- "A large body of clinicopathological, circumstantial, and epidemiological evidence suggests that the **dysregulation** of copper is **intimately** involved in the **pathogenesis** of Alzheimer's disease." [1]
- "Because the general population comes in contact with copper mainly through dietary intake, that is, **food 75%** and **drinking water 25%,** a low-copper diet can reduce the risk of AD in individuals with an altered copper metabolism." [2]
- "The **primary source of such copper is municipal drinking water** and copper found in dietary **supplements**; suggesting that our municipal drinking water should be reversed osmosis and our supplements should essentially be copper free." [3]
- The brain is primarily composed of fat, especially unsaturated fats. The unsaturated fats of the brain are particularly vulnerable to oxidative stress.
  - *Copper significantly accelerates the damage of this tissue.*

96

- Failure of your body to incorporate copper into cerulopasmin (Cp) can at above normal concentrations cross the blood brian barrier producing plaque deposits. [4.]
- "The Environmental Protection Agency (EPA) allows over 10 times (1.3 ppm) that much copper in human drinking water." [4.] [YIKES]
- "The prospective studies revealed an association between a diet simultaneously **high in saturated fatty acids (SFA)** and **Cu** and cognitive decline." [5.]
- "Our meta-analysis results showed that serum **zinc** was **significantly lower** in AD patients. Our replication and meta-analysis results showed that serum **copper** was significantly **higher** in AD patients than in healthy controls, so our findings were consistent with the conclusions of four previously published copper meta-analyses." [7.]
- "…serum **zinc** has been found significantly **decreased** in AD patients compared with healthy controls. [8.]

The Details:

According to:
1. Copper and oxidative stress in the pathogenesis of Alzheimer's disease. Eskici G, Axelsen PH. Biochemistry. 2012 Aug 14;51(32):6289-311. Epub 2012 Jul 31. PMID: 22708607 DOI: 10.1021/bi3006169

"A large body of clinicopathological, circumstantial, and epidemiological evidence suggests that the dysregulation of copper is intimately involved in the pathogenesis of Alzheimer's disease."

According to:
2. Low-copper diet as a preventive strategy for Alzheimer's disease. Squitti R, Siotto M, Polimanti R. et al. Neurobiol Aging. 2014 Sep;35 Suppl 2:S40-50. doi: 10.1016/j.neurobiolaging.2014.02.031. Epub 2014 May 15. PMID: 24913894

"Recent studies have indicated that alteration of copper metabolism is one of the pathogenetic mechanisms of Alzheimer's disease (AD)."

"Because the general population comes in contact with copper mainly through dietary intake, that is, food 75% and drinking water 25%, a low-copper diet can reduce the risk of AD in individuals with an altered copper metabolism."

According to:
3. Oxidative Stress in Alzheimer's Disease and Mild Cognitive Impairment. Natividad Lopez, Consuelo Tormo, Isabel De Blas, et al. Journal of Alzheimer's Disease October 16, 2012 [epub]

Authors Note: damage to cells are called:
- Free Radical Damage
- Oxidative Stress
- Reactive Oxygen Species (ROS)
- Lipid Peroxidation

The brain is primarily composed of fat, especially unsaturated fats. The unsaturated fats of the brain are particularly vulnerable to oxidative stress.

Copper significantly accelerates lipid peroxidation (free radical damage) and is therefore a factor in accelerating mild cognitive impairment (MCI) and Alzheimer's disease.

"The primary source of such copper is municipal drinking water and copper found in dietary supplements; suggesting that our municipal drinking water should be reversed osmosis and our supplements should essentially be copper free."

According to:
4. Low-copper diet as a preventive strategy for Alzheimer's disease. Rosanna Squitti, Mariacristina Siotto, Renato Polimanti. Neurobiology of Aging 2014 epub

"Copper is an essential element, and either a copper deficiency or excess can be life threatening."

"Deficiencies of some micronutrients, especially those related to antioxidant and amino acid metabolism mechanisms (e.g., vitamins B1, B2, B6, B12, C, and folate), have been associated with cognitive impairment in elderly people."

"One of the most recent concepts in AD pathogenesis is that alterations of copper metabolism associated with genetic defects are associated with a 'copper phenotype' in a large percentage of AD patients."

The minimal acceptable intake of copper is about 0.9-1.3 mg per day,whereas, the average person consumes about 2 mg per day. Ingesting 2-3 mg per day of copper is safe and adequately prevents copper deficiency.

Defects in copper homeostasis result in serious health consequences, "specifically for brain health and development."

"An increase in copper levels is established in specific cancers (i.e., breast, cervical, ovarian, lung, prostate, stomach, and leukemia)." The association between increased copper and cancer is likely because of increased oxidative stress causing tumor onset and progression and mitochondrial mutations.

"An increase of 1 mmol/L in total serum copper accounted for 80% of the risk of having AD."

In Alzheimer's disease, copper absorption is normal, but there is a failure in its incorporation into ceruloplasmin (Cp). "This causes an overflow of non-Cp copper sufficiently to be detected in general circulation." When values of non-Cp copper exceed 1.6 mmol/L, it crosses the brain blood barrier (BBB), producing amyloidbeta (Ab) increasing and Ab-plaque deposition.

"We suggest that individuals with high copper-related AD risk should adopt a low copper diet, that is, increase the quantity of low-copper foods, whereas reducing the quantity of high-copper foods, fatty foods, and alcohol consumption (that affects liver functionality). These individuals should also take zinc supplements, provided this can be done under medical supervision."

0.12 ppm (parts per million) of copper added to distilled water trigger Alzheimer's plaques. "The Environmental Protection Agency (EPA) allows over 10 times (1.3 ppm) that much copper in human drinking water."

According to:
5. Copper and iron in Alzheimer's disease: a systematic review and its dietary implications. Loef M1, Walach H. Br J Nutr. 2012 Jan;107(1):7-19. PMID: 21767446 DOI: 10.1017/S000711451100376X Epub 2011 Jul 18.

"To establish the relationship between diets high in Cu and Fe and cognitive decline or AD, we have conducted a systematic review of the literature (up to January 2011)."
"We identified two meta-analyses, two systematic reviews, eleven placebo-controlled trials, five observational studies, forty-five case-control studies, thirty autopsy and five uncontrolled studies, and one case report."

"The prospective studies revealed an association between a diet simultaneously high in SFA and Cu and cognitive decline."

"In conclusion, the existing data suggest that diets excessive in Fe or Cu, together with a high intake of SFA, should be avoided in the elderly who are not at risk of anaemia."

According to:
6. Serum copper in Alzheimer's disease and vascular dementia. Agarwal R, Kushwaha SS, Tripathi CB, et al. Indian J Clin Biochem. 2008 Oct;23(4):369-74. PMID: 23105789 PMCID: PMC3453128 DOI: 10.1007/s12291-008-0081-8 Epub 2008 Dec 20.

"Oxidative stress plays important role in the pathophysiology of Alzheimer's disease. Metals like copper, iron derived through diet can act as pro-oxidant under oxidative stress."

"Our study found weak correlation between copper and ceruloplasmin levels in Alzheimer's disease and Vascular Dementia."

According to:
7. Serum Iron, Zinc, and Copper Levels in Patients with Alzheimer's Disease: A Replication Study and Meta-Analyses. Wang ZX, Tan L, Wang HF, et al. J Alzheimers Dis. 2015;47(3):565-81. doi: 10.3233/JAD-143108. PMID: 26401693 DOI: 10.3233/JAD-143108

"To evaluate whether iron, zinc, and copper levels in serum are disarranged in Alzheimer's disease (AD), we performed meta-analyses of all studies on the topic published from 1984 to 2014 and contextually carried out a replication study in serum as well."

"Our meta-analysis results showed that serum zinc was significantly lower in AD patients. Our replication and meta-analysis results showed that serum copper was significantly higher in AD patients than in healthy controls, so our findings were consistent with the conclusions of four previously published copper meta-analyses."

According to:
8. Zinc and Copper in Alzheimer's Disease. Avan A, Hoogenraad TU. J Alzheimers Dis. 2015;46(1):89-92. doi: 10.3233/JAD-150186. PMID: 25835420 DOI: 10.3233/JAD-150186

"In a recent meta-analysis by Ventriglia and colleagues studying the association of zinc levels with Alzheimer's disease (AD), serum zinc has been found significantly decreased in AD patients compared with healthy controls."

"On the basis of available evidence, free copper toxicosis may play a causal role in age-related AD, and zinc therapy can be a rational causal treatment."

According to:
9. Metal and complementary molecular bioimaging in Alzheimer's disease. Braidy N, Poljak A, Marjo C, et al. Front Aging Neurosci. 2014 Jul 15;6:138. eCollection 2014. PMID: 25076902 PMCID: PMC4098123 DOI: 10.3389/fnagi.2014.00138

"Alzheimer's disease (AD) is the leading cause of dementia in the elderly, affecting over 27 million people worldwide."

"At a molecular level, metal dyshomeostasis is frequently observed in AD due to anomalous binding of metals such as Iron (Fe), Copper (Cu), and Zinc (Zn), or impaired regulation of redox-active metals which can induce the formation of cytotoxic reactive oxygen species and neuronal damage."

Diabetes: ↑

The Short Story:
Defined: A disease that affect how your body uses blood sugar.

Summary: Type 3 diabetes is a title that has been proposed for Alzheimer's disease which results from resistance to insulin in the brain.   So, think of every bite of sugar / carbohydrate as killing parts of your brain!

Lightning facts:
- Diabetes **doubles** the AD risk. [1.]
- "Studies have often shown a 40–50% **reduced** risk of dementia associated with high (omega 3 Fatty Acids) n-3 intake." [1.]
- Exposure to nitrates, nitrites via processed / **preserved food** have critical roles in pathogenesis of our insulin resistance. [2.]
- "In order to effectively halt the process of neurodegeneration, the forces that advance and perpetuate the disease, particularly with regard to the progressive worsening of **brain insulin**/IGF **resistance**, must be understood." [3.]
- "Here we review emerging evidence that **restriction** of dietary advanced glycation end-products **significantly reduces** total systemic load and insulin resistance in animals and humans in diabetes, polycystic ovary syndrome, healthy populations and dementia." [4.]

- "Most children and adults with T1D (type 1 Diabetes) typically manifest lower scores on measures of intelligence and academic achievement, attention, psychomotor speed, and executive functions. These effects are especially pronounced in those who develop diabetes early in life, before the age of 6 or 7 years." [5.]
- "They (T1D) are also at **increased risk** of developing dementia." [5.]
- "The pathophysiology includes defects in insulin signaling, autonomic function, neuroinflammatory pathways, mitochondrial (Mt) metabolism, the sirtuin-peroxisome proliferator-activated receptor-gamma co-activator 1α (SIRT-PGC-1α) axis, and Tau signaling." [6.]
- "There is **strong** evidence that diabetes mellitus **increases** the risk of cognitive impairment and dementia. Insulin signaling dysregulation and small vessel disease in the base of diabetes may be important contributing factors in Alzheimer's disease and vascular dementia pathogenesis, respectively." [7.]
- "The impaired **glucose metabolism in the brain** of subject with AD is a **widely recognized** early feature of the disease; in vivo evaluation with PET is a useful diagnostic tool." [8.]

The Details:

According to:

1. Dietary fatty acids and the aging brain. Greg M Cole, Qiu-Lan Ma, Sally A Frautschy Nutrition Reviews Volume 68, Issue Supplement s2, pages S102–S111, December 2010 Departments of Medicine and Neurology, University of California, Los Angeles

"Nutritional interventions are not only highly relevant to aging in general, they are also inherently more likely to have lower costs and a more favorable safety profile than novel drugs."

Diabetes doubles the AD risk.

"Low n-3 fatty acid intake is one of many overlapping risk factors for both CVD and AD that include type II diabetes, hypercholesterolemia, hypertension, hyperhomo-cysteinemia, dietary saturated fats, cholesterol, low intake of antioxidants, high alcohol consumption, low physical activity or sedentary lifestyle, the presence of atrial fibrillation, and atherosclerotic disease."

"Studies have often shown a 40–50% reduced risk of dementia associated with high n-3 intake."

DHA improves synaptic membrane fluidity, reduces Aâ production by several proposed mechanisms, limits formation of tau pathology/neurofibrillary tangles.

According to:
2. Epidemilogical trends strongly suggest exposures as etiologic agents in the pathogenesis of sporadic Alzheimer's disease, diabetes mellitus, and non-alcoholic steatohepatitis. de la Monte SM, Neusner A, Chu J, Lawton M. J Alzheimers Dis. 2009;17(3):519-29. PMID: 19363256 [PubMed - indexed for MEDLINE]

"Herein, we review evidence that the upwardly spiraling trends in mortality rates due to DM, AD, and Parkinson's disease typify exposure rather than genetic-based disease models, and parallel the progressive increases in human exposure to nitrates, nitrites, and nitrosamines via processed/preserved foods."

"We propose that such chronic exposures have critical roles in the pathogenesis of our insulin resistance disease pandemic. Potential solutions include: 1) eliminating the use of nitrites in food; 2) reducing nitrate levels in fertilizer and water used to irrigate crops; and 3) employing safe and effective measures to detoxify food and water prior to human consumption."

According to:
3. The study, "Dysfunctional Pro-Ceramide, ER Stress, and Insulin/IGF Signaling Networks with Progression of Alzheimer's Disease", is published in the June 22, 2012, supplement of the Journal of Alzheimer's Disease.

"In order to effectively halt the process of neurodegeneration, the forces that advance and perpetuate the disease, particularly with regard to the progressive worsening of brain insulin/IGF resistance, must be understood."

"Brain insulin resistance (diabetes) is very much like regular diabetes," de la Monte said. "Since the underlying problems continue to be just about the same, we believe that the development of new therapies would be applicable for all types of diabetes, including Alzheimer's disease, which we refer to as Type III diabetes."

According to:
4. Advanced glycation end-products: modifiable environmental factors profoundly mediate insulin resistance. Ottum MS, Mistry AM. J Clin Biochem Nutr. 2015 Jul;57(1):1-12. Epub 2015 Jul 1. PMID: 26236094 PMCID: PMC4512899 DOI: 10.3164/jcbn.15-3

"Advanced glycation end-products are toxic by-products of metabolism and are also acquired from high-temperature processed foods. They promote oxidative damage to proteins, lipids and nucleotides."

"High advanced glycation end-products overwhelm innate defenses of enzymes and receptor-mediated endocytosis and promote cell damage via the pro-inflammatory and pro-oxidant receptor for advanced glycation end-products."

"Here we review emerging evidence that restriction of dietary advanced glycation end-products significantly reduces total systemic load and insulin resistance in animals and humans in diabetes, polycystic ovary syndrome, healthy populations and dementia."

According to:
5. Neurocognitive consequences of diabetes.
Ryan CM, van Duinkerken E, Rosano C. Am Psychol.
2016 Oct;71(7):563-576. PMID: 27690485 DOI:
10.1037/a0040455

"Mild cognitive dysfunction is a well-established complication of diabetes and its management, although large numbers of psychologists and health professionals may be unaware of its existence, clinical implications, and etiology."

"Most children and adults with T1D typically manifest lower scores on measures of intelligence and academic achievement, attention, psychomotor speed, and executive functions. These effects are especially pronounced in those who develop diabetes early in life, before the age of 6 or 7 years."

"They are also at increased risk of developing dementia."

6. Diabetes and Cognitive Impairment.
Zilliox LA, Chadrasekaran K, Kwan JY, et al. Curr Diab
Rep. 2016 Sep;16(9):87. doi: 10.1007/s11892-016-0775-x.
PMID: 27491830 DOI: 10.1007/s11892-016-0775-x

"Both type 1 (T1DM) and type 2 diabetes mellitus (T2DM) have been associated with reduced performance on multiple domains of cognitive function and with evidence of abnormal structural and functional brain magnetic resonance imaging (MRI)."

"The pathophysiology includes defects in insulin signaling, autonomic function, neuroinflammatory pathways, mitochondrial (Mt) metabolism, the sirtuin-peroxisome proliferator-activated receptor-gamma co-activator 1α (SIRT-PGC-1α) axis, and Tau signaling."

According to:
7. Diabetes mellitus and cognitive impairments.
Saedi E, Gheini MR, Faiz F, et al. World J Diabetes. 2016 Sep 15;7(17):412-22. PMID: 27660698 PMCID: PMC5027005 DOI: 10.4239/wjd.v7.i17.412

"There is strong evidence that diabetes mellitus increases the risk of cognitive impairment and dementia. Insulin signaling dysregulation and small vessel disease in the base of diabetes may be important contributing factors in Alzheimer's disease and vascular dementia pathogenesis, respectively."

"Anti-diabetic medications especially Insulin may have a role in the management of cognitive dysfunction and dementia but further investigation is needed to validate these findings."

According to:
8. Alterations in glucose metabolism in Alzheimer's disease. Calsolaro V, Edison P. Recent Pat Endocr Metab Immune Drug Discov. 2016 Jun 14. [Epub ahead of print]

"Alzheimer's disease (AD) is the most frequent type of dementia in people over 65 years of age; type 2 diabetes mellitus is a metabolic condition affecting 382 million of adults worldwide."

"In this paper, we discuss how [18F]FDG is a marker of glucose metabolism, how insulin resistance is related to diabetes, the link between diabetes and AD, and how novel treatments for diabetes could be beneficial in the treatment of Alzheimer's disease."

"The impaired glucose metabolism in the brain of subject with AD is a widely recognised early feature of the disease; in vivo evaluation with PET is a useful diagnostic tool. The link between diabetes and neurodegeneration is widely recognized and offer a target for novel therapeutic strategies."

According to:
8. Alterations in Glucose Metabolism on Cognition: A Possible Link Between Diabetes and Dementia. González-Reyes RE, Aliev G, Ávila-Rodrigues M, et al. Curr Pharm Des. 2016;22(7):812-8. PMID: 26648470 [PubMed - in process]

"Any disruption of this physiological balance may result in a dangerous compromise of general metabolic activities increasing the possibility of developing T1DM, T2DM and possibly AD."

"Astrocytes convert glucose into lactate and transfer it to neurons."

"This lactate is essential for neuronal metabolism and for various processes including the formation of synapses, dendrites and the expression of genes involved in memory."

"As the brain ages, it seems to become much more susceptible to cellular damage induced by excess of circulating glucose and this could explain the appearance of cognitive changes observed in some patients with diabetes."

Exercise: ↓

The Short Story:
Defined: There are a lot of definitions but what we are shooting for is physical exercise with the goal of improving health by planned and organized intent.

Summary: Most people know exercise is good but fail to get in due to how busy life can begin. Don't let the business of life push you into a position where you elevate your dementia or Alzheimer's risk.

Lightning facts:
- "Persons who **exercised 3 or more times per week** were **more likely to be dementia-free** than those who exercised fewer than 3 times per week." [1.]
- Home-based exercise tested with sitting Tai Chi for both patient and caregiver helped both: exercise for the dementia patient and less depression for the caregiver. [2.]
- "The effects of exercise and physical activity on cognitive function and brain health have been established by longitudinal and intervention studies." [3.]
- "Exercise may **improve functional** outcomes in Parkinson's disease (PD), and Alzheimer's disease (AD)." [4.]
  - *Note: there is not enough research to determine this on Lewy Body Dementia yet.*

The Details:

According to:

1. Exercise Is Associated with Reduced Risk for Incident Dementia among Persons 65 Years of Age and Older. Eric B. Larson, MD, MPH; Li Wang, et al. Annals Of Internal Medicine January 17, 2006, Volume 144 Issue 2, pp 73-81

"1740 persons older than age 65 years without cognitive impairment."

"During a mean follow-up of 6.2 years, 158 participants developed dementia (107 developed Alzheimer disease). [Scary, this is 9% in 6 years] The incidence rate of dementia was 13.0 per 1000 person-years for participants who exercised 3 or more times per week compared with 19.7 per 1000 person years for those who exercised fewer than 3 times per week."

"These results suggest that regular exercise is associated with a delay in onset of dementia and Alzheimer disease, further supporting its value for elderly persons."

"Persons who exercised 3 or more times per week were more likely to be dementia-free than those who exercised fewer than 3 times per week."

According to:

2. A home-based exercise intervention for caregivers of persons with dementia: study protocol for a randomised controlled trial. Chan WC, Lautenschlager N, Dow B, et al. Trials. 2016 Sep 21;17(1):460.

"Family members, who provide the majority of care for persons with dementia, are especially vulnerable to developing depression. Interventions targeting their depressive symptoms have been proposed but their efficacies vary considerably. It has been suggested that interventions carried out in the home setting and involving both caregivers and care recipients are more efficacious."

"A total of 136 caregiver-care-recipient dyads (i.e. 272 participants in total) will be recruited and randomly allocated to either a home-based structured exercise (sitting Tai Chi) group or a social contact control group."

"The findings offer a potential avenue of intervention by providing a low-cost, safe and effective treatment for depression among dementia caregivers, which may in turn also benefit the care recipients."

According to:
3. [Exercise and Physical Activity for Dementia Prevention]. [Article in Japanese] Shimada H, Makizako H, Doi T. Brain Nerve. 2016 Jul;68(7):799-808. PMID: 27395464 DOI: 10.11477/mf.1416200512

"The effects of exercise and physical activity on cognitive function and brain health have been established by longitudinal and intervention studies."

"It is also important to identify the adequate duration, frequency, and intensity of exercise intervention that is most effective for older individuals."

According to:

4. Exercise for Individuals with Lewy Body Dementia: A Systematic Review. Inskip M, Mavros Y, Sachdev PS, et al. PLoS One. 2016 Jun 3;11(6):e0156520. eCollection 2016. PMID: 27258533 PMCID: PMC4892610 DOI: 10.1371/journal.pone.0156520

"Individuals with Lewy body Dementia (LBD), which encompasses both Parkinson disease dementia (PDD) and Dementia with Lewy Bodies (DLB) experience functional decline through Parkinsonism and sedentariness exacerbated by motor, psychiatric and cognitive symptoms."

"Exercise may improve functional outcomes in Parkinson's disease (PD), and Alzheimer's disease (AD)."

"Scarce research investigating exercise in LBD exists. This review confirms exercise studies in PD and dementia consistently exclude LBD participants."

Fish: ↓

The Short Story:
Defined: The meat from fish.

Summary: **Eat more fish** and less sweets, fried potatoes, high-fat dairies, processed meat and butter.

Lightning facts:
- "For example, when Japan made the nutrition transition from the traditional Japanese diet to the Western diet, AD rates **rose from 1% in 1985 to 7% in 2008.**" [1.]
- "In cross-sectional analyses, **moderate** seafood consumption was correlated with **lesser** Alzheimer disease neuropathology." [2.]
- Diet affects dementia: [3.]
  - **Decrease** dementia by:
    - 16% with Unsaturated Fatty Acids
    - 13% with antioxidants,
    - 28% with vitamin B
    - 31% with Mediterranean diet
  - **Increase** dementia by:
    - 224% with aluminum
    - 43% with smoking
    - 152% with low Vitamin D
- "'AD-protective' nutrient combination was associated with **higher** intake of fresh fruit and vegetables, whole grains, fish and low-fat dairies, and **lower** intake of sweets, fried potatoes, high-fat dairies, processed meat and butter." [4.]

118

- "If the **onset** of AD can be reduced by as little as one year, the **prevalence** could be **reduced by 10%.**" [5.]
- Those who ate fatty fish **1xweek** decrease Alzheimer's by **60%**!

The Details:
According to:
1. Using Multicountry Ecological and Observational Studies to Determine Dietary Risk Factors for Alzheimer's Disease. Grant WB. J Am Coll Nutr. 2016 Jul;35(5):476-89. PMID: 27454859 DOI: 10.1080/07315724.2016.1161566

The most important risk factors to the quick rise of Alzheimer's Disease seem to be linked to diet.

"For example, when Japan made the nutrition transition from the traditional Japanese diet to the Western diet, AD rates rose from 1% in 1985 to 7% in 2008."

"Foods protective against AD include fruits, vegetables, grains, low-fat dairy products, legumes, and fish, whereas risk factors include meat, sweets, and high-fat dairy products."

"Lower 25-hydroxyvitamin D concentrations also are associated with increased risk of AD."

"Thus, reducing meat consumption could significantly reduce the risk of AD as well as of several cancers, diabetes mellitus type 2, stroke, and, likely, chronic kidney disease."

According to:
2. Association of Seafood Consumption, Brain Mercury Level, and APOE ε4 Status With Brain Neuropathology in Older Adults. Morris MC, Brockman J, Schneider JA, et al. JAMA. 2016 Feb 2;315(5):489-97. PMID: 26836731 DOI: 10.1001/jama.2015.19451

"Seafood consumption is promoted for its many health benefits even though its contamination by mercury, a known neurotoxin, is a growing concern."

"Cross-sectional analyses of deceased participants in the Memory and Aging Project clinical neuropathological cohort study, 2004-2013. Participants resided in Chicago retirement communities and subsidized housing. The study included 286 autopsied brains of 554 deceased participants (51.6%). The mean (SD) age at death was 89.9 (6.1) years, 67% (193) were women, and the mean (SD) educational attainment was 14.6 (2.7) years."

"In cross-sectional analyses, moderate seafood consumption was correlated with lesser Alzheimer disease neuropathology. Although seafood consumption was also correlated with higher brain levels of mercury, these levels were not correlated with brain neuropathology."

According to:
3. Dietary Patterns and Risk of Dementia: a Systematic Review and Meta-Analysis of Cohort Studies. Cao L, Tan L, Wang HF, et al. Mol Neurobiol. 2015 Nov 9. PMID: 26553347 DOI: 10.1007/s12035-015-9516-4

"Finally, there were 43 trials that met the inclusion standard."

"Dietary patterns and some dietary components have been linked with dementia. We therefore performed a meta-analysis of available studies to determine whether there is an association between diet and risk of dementia."

"Some food intake was related with decrease of dementia, such as unsaturated fatty acids (RR: 0.84, 95 % CI: [0.74-0.95], P = 0.006), antioxidants (RR: 0.87, 95 % CI: [0.77-0.98], P = 0.026), vitamin B (RR: 0.72, 95 % CI: [0.54-0.96], P = 0.026), and the Mediterranean diet (MeDi) (RR: 0.69, 95 % CI: [0.57-0.84], P < 0.001)."

"Some material intakes were related with increase of dementia, such as aluminum (RR: 2.24, 95 % CI: [1.49-3.37], P < 0.001), smoking (RR: 1.43, 95 % CI: [1.15-1.77], P = 0.001), and low levels of vitamin D (RR: 1.52, 95 % CI: [1.17-1.98], P = 0.002)."

According to:
4. Nutrient patterns and brain biomarkers of Alzheimer's disease in cognitively normal individuals. Berti V, Murray J, Davies M, Spector N, et al. J Nutr Health Aging. 2015 Apr;19(4):413-23. PMID: 25809805 PMCID: PMC4375781 DOI: 10.1007/s12603-014-0534-0

"This study identifies nutrient patterns associated with major brain AD biomarkers in a cohort of clinically and cognitively normal (NL) individuals at risk for AD."

"None of the participants were diabetics, smokers, or met criteria for obesity."

"Five NPs (neuroprotective) were identified: NP1 was characterized by most B-vitamins and several minerals [VitB and Minerals]; NP2 by monounsaturated and polyunsaturated fats, including ω-3 and ω-6 PUFA, and vitamin E [VitE and PUFA]; NP3 by vitamin A, vitamin C, carotenoids and dietary fibers [Anti-oxidants and Fibers]; NP4 by vitamin B12, vitamin D and zinc [VitB12 and D]; NP5 by saturated, trans-saturated fats, cholesterol and sodium [Fats]."

"The identified 'AD-protective' nutrient combination was associated with higher intake of fresh fruit and vegetables, whole grains, fish and low-fat dairies, and lower intake of sweets, fried potatoes, high-fat dairies, processed meat and butter."

According to:
5. Consumption of fish and Alzheimer's disease. Newton W, McManus A. J Nutr Health Aging. 2011 Aug;15(7):551-4552. PMID: 21808933

"Based on the current prevalence of AD, an aging world population and the associated projected health care requirements, it is estimated that by 2050, the prevalence of AD will reach 104 million with around 43% requiring ongoing health care."

"If the onset of AD can be reduced by as little as one year, the prevalence could be reduced by 10%."

"There is substantial commonality in research findings to date around the positive influence of seafood consumption in reducing the risk of dementia and AD."

According to:
6. Fish, meat, and risk of dementia: cohort study. Pascale Barberger-Gateau, Luc Letenneur, Valérie Deschamps, et al. British Medical Journal, Vol. 325, October 26, 2002, pg 932-933

Fatty acids could be involved in dementia through these mechanisms:
(1) Atherosclerosis
(2) Thrombosis
(3) Inflammation

Consumption of n-3 fatty acids by eating fish once per week significantly reduce the risk of dementia and Alzheimer's Disease.

Eating red meat does not increase the risk of dementia or Alzheimer's Disease.

Those who ate fatty fish 1xweek decrease Alzheimer's by 60%!

Fish Oil (Omega 3 &DHA): ↓

The Short Story:

Defined: A oil extracted from fish under controlled and purified constraints.

Summary: Simple: Take fish oil, specifically a special extracted form called DHA. Such a tiny dose (0.1-g/d) increment of dietary docosahexaenoic acid (DHA) intake was associated with **lower** risks of dementia!!

Lightning facts:

- "In one study, consumption of preformed DHA was **7 times more likely** to result in uptake by the brain than DHA derived through consumption of linolenic acid." [1.]
- "FOS use during follow-up was associated with **significantly lower** mean cognitive subscale of the Alzheimer's Disease Assessment Scale and higher Mini-Mental State Examination scores among those with normal cognition." [2.]
- "Participants who consumed fish **once per week** or more had **60% less risk** of Alzheimer disease compared with those who rarely or never ate fish in a model adjusted for age and other risk factors." [4.]

- "Nutrients examined included saturated fatty acid, monounsaturated fatty acid, ω-3 polyunsaturated fatty acid (PUFA), ω-6 PUFA, **vitamin E, vitamin C, β-carotene, vitamin B(12), folate, and vitamin D**." [3.]
    o This lead to a **reduced risk** of incident AD and slower cognitive decline in our cohort.
- "DHA is **essential** for brain **development** and function." [5.]
- "We included 21 studies (181,580 participants) with 4438 cases identified during follow-up periods (2.1-21 y). [6.]
    o 1-serving/wk increment of dietary fish was associated with lower risks of:
        - Dementia lower by 5%
        - AD lower by 7%
- "Mechanistic studies, epidemiologic analyses, and randomized controlled intervention trials provide insight to the **positive effects** of docosahexaenoic acid (DHA) and micronutrients such as the vitamin **B family, and vitamins E, C, and D**, in helping neurons to cope with aging." [7.]
- "Our study shows that DHA plays a role in **mitigating** AβPP-induced impairment in energy metabolism and **inflammation** by acting on tricarboxylic acid cycle, cholesterol biosynthesis pathway and fatty acid metabolism." [8.]

The Details:
According to:
1. Consumption of Fish and n-3 Fatty Acids and Risk of Incident Alzheimer Disease. Martha Clare Morris, ScD; Denis A. Evans, MD; Julia L. Bienias, et al. Archives of Neurology; Vol. 60 No. 7; pp. 940-946; July 2003

"Docosahexaenoic acid is selectively accumulated in the brain during fetal and infant brain growth."

"In one study, consumption of preformed DHA was 7 times more likely to result in uptake by the brain than DHA derived through consumption of linolenic acid."

According to:
2. Association of fish oil supplement use with preservation of brain volume and cognitive function. Daiello LA, Gongvatana A, Dunsiger S, et al. Alzheimers Dement. 2015 Feb;11(2):226-35. Epub 2014 Jun 18. Alzheimer's Disease Neuroimaging Initiative. PMID: 24954371 doi: 10.1016/j.jalz.2014.02.005.

"The aim of this study was to investigate whether the use of fish oil supplements (FOSs) is associated with concomitant reduction in cognitive decline and brain atrophy in older adults."

"Older adults (229 cognitively normal individuals, 397 patients with mild cognitive impairment, and 193 patients with Alzheimer's disease) were assessed with neuropsychological tests and brain magnetic resonance imaging every 6 months."

"FOS use during follow-up was associated with significantly lower mean cognitive subscale of the Alzheimer's Disease Assessment Scale and higher Mini-Mental State Examination scores among those with normal cognition."

"Associations between FOS use and the outcomes were observed only in APOE ε4-negative participants."

According to:
3 Nutrient intake and plasma β-amyloid. Gu Y, Schupf N, Cosentino SA, et al. Neurology. 2012 Jun 5;78(23):1832-40. doi: 10.1212/WNL.0b013e318258f7c2. Epub 2012 May 2. PMID: 22551728 PMCID: PMC3369517 DOI: 10.1212/WNL.0b013e318258f7c2

"The widely reported associations between various nutrients and cognition may occur through many biologic pathways including those of β-amyloid (Aβ)."

"Nutrients examined included saturated fatty acid, monounsaturated fatty acid, ω-3 polyunsaturated fatty acid (PUFA), ω-6 PUFA, vitamin E, vitamin C, β-carotene, vitamin B(12), folate, and vitamin D."

"Our data suggest that higher dietary intake of ω-3 PUFA is associated with lower plasma levels of Aβ42, a profile linked with reduced risk of incident AD and slower cognitive decline in our cohort."

According to:
4. Consumption of fish and n-3 fatty acids and risk of incident Alzheimer disease. Morris MC, Evans DA, Bienias JL, et al. Arch Neurol. 2003 Jul;60(7):940-6. PMID: 12873849 DOI: 10.1001/archneur.60.7.940

"Dietary n-3 polyunsaturated fatty acids improve brain functioning in animal studies, but there is limited study of whether this type of fat protects against Alzheimer disease."

"Prospective study conducted from 1993 through 2000, of a stratified random sample from a geographically defined community. Participants were followed up for an average of 3.9 years for the development of Alzheimer disease."

"Participants who consumed fish once per week or more had 60% less risk of Alzheimer disease compared with those who rarely or never ate fish (relative risk, 0.4; 95% confidence interval, 0.2-0.9) in a model adjusted for age and other risk factors."

"Dietary intake of n-3 fatty acids and weekly consumption of fish may reduce the risk of incident Alzheimer disease."

According to:
5. Docosahexaenoic acid: one molecule diverse functions. Hashimoto M, Hossain S, Al Mamun A,et al. Crit Rev Biotechnol. 2016 Jul 17:1-19. [Epub ahead of print] PMID: 27426008 DOI: 10.1080/07388551.2016.1207153

"Docosahexaenoic acid (DHA, C22:6, ω-3) is a highly polyunsaturated omega-3 fatty acid. It is concentrated in neuronal brain membranes, for which reason it is also referred to as a "brain food"."

"DHA is essential for brain development and function."

"For example, DHA, which inherently has a characteristic three-dimensional structure, increases membrane fluidity, strengthens antioxidant activity and enhances the expression of several proteins that act as substrates for improving memory functions."

"It reduces the brain amyloid burden and inhibits in vitro fibrillation and amyloid-induced neurotoxicity in cell-culture model."

According to:
6. Intakes of fish and polyunsaturated fatty acids and mild-to-severe cognitive impairment risks: a dose-response meta-analysis of 21 cohort studies. Zhang Y, Chen J, Qiu J, et al. Am J Clin Nutr. 2016 Feb;103(2):330-40. doi: 10.3945/ajcn.115.124081. Epub 2015 Dec 30. PMID: 26718417 DOI: 10.3945/ajcn.115.124081

"We systematically investigated associations between fish and PUFA intake and mild-to-severe cognitive impairment risk."

"Studies that reported risk estimates for mild cognitive impairment (MCI), cognitive decline, dementia, Alzheimer disease (AD), or Parkinson disease (PD) from fish, total PUFAs, total n-3 (ω-3) PUFAs, or at least one n-3 PUFA were included."

"We included 21 studies (181,580 participants) with 4438 cases identified during follow-up periods (2.1-21 y). A 1-serving/wk increment of dietary fish was associated with lower risks of dementia (RR: 0.95; 95% CI: 0.90, 0.99; P = 0.042, I(2) = 63.4%) and AD (RR: 0.93; 95% CI: 0.90, 0.95; P = 0.003, I(2) = 74.8%)."

"Pooled RRs of MCI and PD were 0.71 (95% CI: 0.59, 0.82; P = 0.733, I(2) = 0%) and 0.90 (95% CI: 0.80, 0.99; P = 0.221, I(2) = 33.7%), respectively, for an 8-g/d increment of PUFA intake."

"As an important source of marine n-3 PUFAs, a 0.1-g/d increment of dietary docosahexaenoic acid (DHA) intake was associated with lower risks of dementia (RR: 0.86; 95% CI: 0.76, 0.96; P < 0.001, I(2) = 92.7%) and AD (RR: 0.63; 95% CI: 0.51, 0.76; P < 0.001, I(2) = 94.5%)."

According to:
7. Inadequate supply of vitamins and DHA in the elderly: implications for brain aging and Alzheimer-type dementia. Mohajeri MH, Troesch B, Weber P. Nutrition. 2015 Feb;31(2):261-75. Epub 2014 Jul 24. PMID: 25592004 DOI: 10.1016/j.nut.2014.06.016

"Mechanistic studies, epidemiologic analyses, and randomized controlled intervention trials provide insight to the positive effects of docosahexaenoic acid (DHA) and micronutrients such as the vitamin B family, and vitamins E, C, and D, in helping neurons to cope with aging."

"These nutrients are inexpensive in use, have virtually no side effects when used at recommended doses, are essential for life, have established modes of action, and are broadly accepted by the general public."

"This review provides some evidence that the use of vitamins and DHA for the aging population in general, and for individuals at risk in particular, is a viable alternative approach to delaying brain aging and for protecting against the onset of AD pathology."

According to:
8. Metabotyping of docosahexaenoic acid - treated Alzheimer's disease cell model. Bahety P, Tan YM, Hong Y, et al. PLoS One. 2014 Feb 27;9(2):e90123. eCollection 2014. PMID: 24587236 PMCID: PMC3937442 DOI: 10.1371/journal.pone.0090123

"A list of statistically significant marker metabolites that characterized the metabotypes associated with DHA treatment was further identified. Increased levels of succinic acid, citric acid, malic acid and glycine and decreased levels of zymosterol, cholestadiene and arachidonic acid correlated with DHA treatment effect."

"Our study shows that DHA plays a role in mitigating AβPP-induced impairment in energy metabolism and inflammation by acting on tricarboxylic acid cycle, cholesterol biosynthesis pathway and fatty acid metabolism."

Free Radicals: ↑

The Short Story:
Defined: When a molecule has one or more unpaired electrons in the outer shell, thus becoming highly unstable and reactive with normal cells.

Summary: The unsaturated fats of the brain are particularly vulnerable to oxidative stress (free radicle damage). This process is called lipid peroxidation.

Lightning facts:
- "Because of their **selective vulnerability**, these neurons are usually the **first** to exhibit functional **decline** and cell death during normal aging, or in age-associated neurodegenerative diseases, such as Alzheimer's disease." [1.]
- Eat foods **high** in **polyphenolic compounds** as they can **stop free radicals** and **raise** things to **help** protect your brain. [2.]
- There is a relationship between "the influence of free radicals on development of AD and antioxidants as potential drugs toward AD." [5.]
  - So **eat foods rich in antioxidants** like:
    - Blueberries
    - Dark Chocolate
    - Pecans
    - Kidney, Pinto or Black Beans
    - Cranberries
    - Prunes

The Details:

According to:

1. Selective Neuronal Vulnerability to Oxidative Stress in the Brain. Xinkun Wang, and Elias K. Michaelis. Front Aging Neurosci. 2010; 2: 12. Published online 2010 Mar 30. Prepublished online 2010 Jan 6. doi: 10.3389/fnagi.2010.00012 PMCID: PMC2874397

"Oxidative stress (OS), caused by the imbalance between the generation and detoxification of reactive oxygen and nitrogen species (ROS/RNS), plays an important role in brain aging, neurodegenerative diseases, and other related adverse conditions, such as ischemia."

"While ROS/RNS serve as signaling molecules at physiological levels, an excessive amount of these molecules leads to oxidative modification and, therefore, dysfunction of proteins, nucleic acids, and lipids."

"While many brain neurons can cope with a rise in OS, there are select populations of neurons in the brain that are vulnerable."

"Because of their selective vulnerability, these neurons are usually the first to exhibit functional decline and cell death during normal aging, or in age-associated neurodegenerative diseases, such as Alzheimer's disease."

"The contribution to the selective vulnerability of neurons to OS by other intrinsic or extrinsic factors, such as deficient DNA damage repair, low calcium-buffering capacity, and glutamate excitotoxicity, are also discussed."

According to:
2. Dietary Polyphenols as Potential Remedy for Dementia. Desai A1. Adv Neurobiol. 2016;12:41-56. PMID: 27651247 DOI: 10.1007/978-3-319-28383-8_3

"Many processes that are associated with the pathophysiology of dementia can be modulated by polyphenols."

"Polyphenolic compounds can alleviate oxidative stress by acting as direct scavengers of free radicals and clearing superoxide and hydroxyl radicals and by increasing the level of antioxidant enzymes such as glutathione peroxidase."

"The cognitive decline in dementia due to decreased availability of acetylcholine can also be countered by polyphenols that inhibit acetyl-cholinesterase activity."

According to:
3. Role of oxidative stress in Alzheimer's disease.Huang WJ1, Zhang X1, Chen WW1. Biomed Rep. 2016 May;4(5):519-522. Epub 2016 Mar 15. PMID: 27123241 PMCID: PMC4840676 DOI: 10.3892/br.2016.630

"AD is characterized by the abnormal deposition of amyloid β (Aβ) peptide, and intracellular accumulation of neurofibrillary tangles of hyperphosphorylated τ protein and dementia."

"This imbalance can occur as a result of increased free radicals or a decrease in antioxidant defense, free radicals being a species that contains one or more unpaired electrons in its outer shell."

"The major source of potent free radicals is the reduction of molecular oxygen in water, that initially yields the superoxide radical, which produces hydrogen peroxide by the addition of an electron."

"Thus, tissues and organs, particularly the brain, a vulnerable organ, are affected by ROS due to its composition."

According to:
4. Getting to NO Alzheimer's Disease: Neuroprotection versus Neurotoxicity Mediated by Nitric Oxide. Balez R, Ooi L. Oxid Med Cell Longev. 2016;2016:3806157. Epub 2015 Nov 30. PMID: 26697132 PMCID: PMC4677236 DOI: 10.1155/2016/3806157

"Nitric oxide (NO) has long been considered part of the neurotoxic insult caused by neuroinflammation in the Alzheimer's brain."

"This has highlighted a compensatory, neuroprotective role for NO that protects synapses by increasing neuronal excitability."

"Harnessing the protective role of NO and related signaling pathways could provide a therapeutic avenue that prevents synapse loss early in disease."

According to:

5. The influence of common free radicals and antioxidants on development of Alzheimer's Disease. Wojtunik-Kulesza KA, Oniszczuk A, Oniszczuk T, et al. Biomed Pharmacother. 2016 Mar;78:39-49. Epub 2016 Jan 11. PMID: 26898423 DOI: 10.1016/j.biopha.2015.12.024

"Numerous studies have shown several causes of the disorder, one of the most important being oxidative stress."

"Oxidative stress is connected with a disturbance between the levels of free radicals and antioxidants in organisms."

"This review article presents the most important studies connected with the influence of free radicals on development of AD and antioxidants as potential drugs toward AD."

Fruit: ↓

The Short Story:
Defined: A seed bearing structure of food.

Summary: Most of the research says eating berries is where the benefits are.   Blue, black, red…. Eat them often to **reduce** your dementia risk by up to 2.5 years!!

Lightning facts:
- "The findings suggest **that higher fruit and vegetable consumption** may **reduce the risk** of dementia, *especially* among women and those with angina pectoris in midlife." [1.]
- **Berry** intake appears to **delay** cognitive aging by **up to 2.5 years** and **slower rates of cognitive decline.** [2.]
- Berry intake help with: [4.]
    - **Improved** paired associate learning
    - Word list recall
    - Reduced **depressive** symptoms
    - Lower **glucose** levels
- "In that report, participants who ate **larger** quantities blueberries and strawberries had a **lower** likelihood of becoming demented over several years." [5.]
- "Exercise, statin, and **fruit intake** were associated with **lower** risk for AD mortality." [6.]

- "Recent clinical research has demonstrated that **berry fruits** can **prevent** age-related neurodegenerative diseases and **improve** motor and cognitive functions." [8.]

The Details:
According to:
1. Midlife fruit and vegetable consumption and risk of dementia in later life in Swedish twins. Hughes TF, Andel R, Small BJ, Borenstein AR, et al. Am J Geriatr Psychiatry. 2010 May;18(5):413-20. doi: 10.1097/JGP.0b013e3181c65250.

"The authors examined the association between fruit and vegetable consumption in midlife and risk for all types of dementia and AD."

"Participants were 3,779 members of the Swedish Twin Registry who completed a diet questionnaire approximately 30 years before cognitive screening and full clinical evaluation for dementia as part of the study of dementia in Swedish Twins (HARMONY) study."

"The findings suggest that higher fruit and vegetable consumption may reduce the risk of dementia, especially among women and those with angina pectoris in midlife."

According to:
2. Dietary intakes of berries and flavonoids in relation to cognitive decline. Elizabeth E. Devore ScD,*, Jae Hee Kang ScD, Monique M. B. Breteler MD, PhD, et al. Article first published online: 25 APR 2012 DOI: 10.1002/ana.23594

"Beginning in 1980, a semiquantitative food frequency questionnaire was administered every 4 years to Nurses' Health Study participants."

"Using multivariate-adjusted, mixed linear regression, we estimated mean differences in slopes of cognitive decline by long-term berry and flavonoid intakes."

"… indicating that berry intake appears to delay cognitive aging by up to 2.5 years. Additionally, in further supporting evidence, greater intakes of anthocyanidins and total flavonoids were associated with slower rates of cognitive decline."

According to:
3. A berry thought-provoking idea: the potential role of plant polyphenols in the treatment of age-related cognitive disorders. Cherniack EP. Br J Nutr. 2012 Sep;108(5):794-800. Epub 2012 Apr 5. PMID: 22475317 [PubMed - indexed for MEDLINE]

"The metabolic syndrome and its individual components induce a proinflammatory state that damages blood vessels. This condition of chronic inflammation may damage the vasculature of the brain or be directly neurotoxic."

"Published trials of the benefits of grape and blueberry juice in the treatment of small numbers of cognitively impaired persons have recently appeared."

"A grape polyphenol found in grapes, resveratrol, now being studied in humans, and one in grapes and blueberries, pterostilbene, have been found to improve cognition in rodents."

According to:
4. Blueberry supplementation improves memory in older adults. Krikorian R, Shidler MD, Nash TA, et al. J Agric Food Chem. 2010 Apr 14;58(7):3996-4000. doi: 10.1021/jf9029332. PMID: 20047325 [PubMed - indexed for MEDLINE] PMCID: PMC2850944

"Blueberries contain polyphenolic compounds, most prominently anthocyanins, which have antioxidant and anti-inflammatory effects."

"In addition, anthocyanins have been associated with increased neuronal signaling in brain centers, mediating memory function as well as improved glucose disposal, benefits that would be expected to mitigate neurodegeneration."

"At 12 weeks, improved paired associate learning ($p = 0.009$) and word list recall ($p = 0.04$) were observed. In addition, there were trends suggesting reduced depressive symptoms ($p = 0.08$) and lower glucose levels ($p = 0.10$)."

According to:
5. A plant-tastic treatment for cognitive disorders. Cherniack EP. Maturitas. 2012 Aug;72(4):265-6. doi: 10.1016/j.maturitas.2012.05.001. Epub 2012 May 31. PMID: 22658645 [PubMed - indexed for MEDLINE]

"In that report, participants who ate larger quantities blueberries and strawberries had a lower likelihood of becoming demented over several years."

"Finally, an association was found between trend to greater impairment in cognition and total consumption of anthocyanidins, pigment-conferring polyphenols found in many different plants, such as blueberries and eggplants."

"Berries are packed with various phytochemicals, but the most notable is a large class of polyphenols, of which phenolic acids and flavonoids are members, which are potent antioxidant/anti-inflammatory substances in nature."

" A subset of flavonois, called anthocyanidins, not only has the potency to discharge or negate free radical effects in the brain, but also has been demonstrated to affect intraneural signaling and inhibid lipid peroxidation and the inflammatory mediators Cox-1 and 2."

According to:
6. Lower risk of Alzheimer's disease mortality with exercise, statin, and fruit intake. Williams PT. J Alzheimers Dis. 2015;44(4):1121-9. doi: 10.3233/JAD-141929. PMID: 25408208 DOI: 10.3233/JAD-141929

"Test whether exercise, diet, or statins affect AD mortality in 153,536 participants of the National Runners' and Walkers' Health Studies."

"Relative to exercising <1.07 MET-hours/d, AD mortality was 6.0% lower for 1.07 to 1.8 MET-hours/d (HR: 0.94, 95% CI: 0.59 to 1.46, p = 0.79), 24.8% lower for 1.8 to 3.6 MET-hours/d (HR: 0.75, 95% CI: 0.50 to 1.13, p = 0.17), and 40.1% lower for ≥3.6 MET-hours/d (HR: 0.60, 95% CI: 0.37 to 0.97, p = 0.04). Relative to non-use, statin use was associated with 61% lower AD mortality (HR: 0.39, 95% CI: 0.15 to 0.82, p = 0.01), whereas use of other cholesterol-lowering medications was not (HR: 0.78, 95% CI: 0.40 to 1.38, p = 0.42). Relative to <1 piece of fruit/day, consuming 2 to 3 pieces daily was associated with 39.7% lower AD mortality (HR: 0.60, 95% CI: 0.39 to 0.91, p = 0.02) and ≥3 pieces/day with 60.7% lower AD mortality (HR: 0.39, 95% CI: 0.22 to 0.67, p = 0.0004)."

"Exercise, statin, and fruit intake were associated with lower risk for AD mortality."

According to:
7. Berries: anti-inflammatory effects in humans. Joseph SV, Edirisinghe I, Burton-Freeman BM. J Agric Food Chem. 2014 May 7;62(18):3886-903. doi: 10.1021/jf4044056. Epub 2014 Mar 17. PMID: 24512603 DOI: 10.1021/jf4044056

"Fruits, such as berries, contain polyphenol compounds purported to have anti-inflammatory activity in humans."

"Berries have been studied widely for their antioxidant properties; however, preclinical data suggest important effects on inflammatory pathways."

According to:
8. Neuroprotective effects of berry fruits on neurodegenerative diseases. Subash S, Essa MM, Al-Adawi S, et al. Neural Regen Res. 2014 Aug 15;9(16):1557-66. PMID: 25317174 PMCID: PMC4192974 DOI: 10.4103/1673-5374.139483

"Recent clinical research has demonstrated that berry fruits can prevent age-related neurodegenerative diseases and improve motor and cognitive functions."

"The berry fruits are also capable of modulating signaling pathways involved in inflammation, cell survival, neurotransmission and enhancing neuroplasticity."

"The neuroprotective effects of berry fruits on neurodegenerative diseases are related to phytochemicals such as anthocyanin, caffeic acid, catechin, quercetin, kaempferol and tannin."

According to:
9. Preserving Brain Function in Aging: The Anti-glycative Potential of Berry Fruit. Thangthaeng N, Poulose SM, Miller MG, et al. Neuromolecular Med. 2016 Sep;18(3):465-73. Epub 2016 May 11. PMID: 27166828 DOI: 10.1007/s12017-016-8400-3

"In the diet, Advanced glycation end products (AGEs) are found in animal products, and additional AGEs are produced when those foods are cooked at high temperatures."

"Emerging evidence has shown that the phytochemicals found in berry fruits exhibit anti-glycative activity."

Ginger: ↓

The Short Story:
Defined: A spice made from the ginger plant.

Summary: Eating ginger or ginger extracts helps **decrease** Alzheimer's Disease. This product has been used for centuries in S. Asia to treat dementia.

Lightning facts:
- Ginger is a promising candidate for the **treatment** of Alzheimer's Disease. [1]
- Ginger is a **highly promising** therapeutic compound against AD. [2]
- **Dried ginger** works against two processes (Calcium antagonist and BuChE inhibition) which will **benefit** dementia and AD. [3]

The Details:
According to:
1. Ginger components as new leads for the design and development of novel multi-targeted anti-Alzheimer's drugs: a computational investigation. Azam F, Amer AM, Abulifa AR, et al. Drug Des Devel Ther. 2014 Oct 23;8:2045-59. eCollection 2014. PMID: 25364231 PMCID: PMC4211852 DOI: 10.2147/DDDT.S67778

"Therefore, the present study seeks to employ molecular docking studies to investigate the binding interactions between active ginger components and various anti-Alzheimer drug targets."

"In addition, drug-likeness score and molecular properties responsible for a good pharmacokinetic profile were calculated by Osiris property explorer and Molinspiration online toolkit, respectively. None of the compounds violated Lipinski's rule of five, making them potentially promising drug candidates for the treatment of Alzheimer's disease."

According to:
2. Brain Food for Alzheimer-Free Ageing: Focus on Herbal Medicines. Hügel HM. Adv Exp Med Biol. 2015;863:95-116. PMID: 26092628 DOI: 10.1007/978-3-319-18365-7_5

"Beyond 60 years of age, most, if not everyone, will experience a decline in cognitive skills, memory capacity and changes in brain structure."

"Longevity eventually leads to an accumulation of amyloid plaques and/or tau tangles, including some vascular dementia damage."

"Plants can be considered as chemical factories that manufacture huge numbers of diverse bioactive substances, many of which have the potential to provide substantial neuroprotective benefits."

"Many herbs with anti-amyloidogenic activity, including those containing polyphenolic constituents such as green tea, turmeric, Salvia miltiorrhiza, and Panax ginseng, are presented."

"Also covered in this review are extracts from kitchen spices including cinnamon, ginger, rosemary, sage, salvia herbs, Chinese celery and many others some of which are commonly used in herbal combinations and represent highly promising therapeutic natural compounds against AD."

According to:
3. Muscarinic, Ca(++) antagonist and specific butyrylcholinesterase inhibitory activity of dried ginger extract might explain its use in dementia. Ghayur MN, Gilani AH, Ahmed T, Khalid A, et al. J Pharm Pharmacol. 2008 Oct;60(10):1375-83. PMID: 18812031 DOI: 10.1211/jpp/60.10.0014

"Ginger rhizome (Zingiber officinale) has been used for centuries to treat dementia in South Asia."

"Zo.Cr tested positive for the presence of terpenoids, flavonoids, secondary amines, phenols, alkaloids and saponins."

"This study shows a unique combination of muscarinic, possible Ca(++) antagonist and BuChE inhibitory activities of dried ginger, indicating its benefit in dementia, including Alzheimer's disease."

Gingko Biloba: ↓

<u>The Short Story:</u>
Defined: Ginkgo biloba is a medicine / supplement made from the leaves of the Ginkgo Tree.

Summary: Take 240 mg/day of **EGb 761** supplement that has been around for over 30 years!

Lightning facts:
- Gingko Biloba is one of several to help **slow** AD. [1.]
- "Ginkgo biloba is **potentially** beneficial for the **improvement** of cognitive function, activities of daily living, and global clinical assessment in patients with **mild** cognitive impairment or Alzheimer's disease." [2.]
- "The standardized Ginkgo biloba **extract EGb 761** was marketed in France and Germany **30 years ago** for various vascular and cerebral deficits and is now classified as a food supplement in the United States." [4.]
- "EGb 761® **improved** cognitive functioning, neuropsychiatric symptoms and functional abilities in both types of dementia." [3.]
- "Taking a **240-mg daily** dose of Ginkgo biloba extract is effective and safe in the treatment of dementia." [5.]

- "**EGb761 at 240 mg/day** is able to **stabilize** or **slow decline** in cognition, function, behavior, and global change at 22-26 weeks in cognitive impairment and dementia, especially for patients with neuropsychiatric symptoms." [7.]

The Details:
According to:
1. Influence of the severity of cognitive impairment on the effect of the Ginkgo biloba extract EGb 761 in Alzheimer's disease. Le Bars PL, Velasco FM, Ferguson JM, et al. Neuropsychobiology 2002; 45: 19-26

"Treatment with 600 mg of alpha-lipoic acid daily for 337 days led to a stabilization of cognitive function, in a group of AD and other dementia patients."

"Others have noted cognitive improvement with supplementation of 3-8 g/day of thiamine."

The following antioxidants slow the progression of Alzheimer's disease:
- Vitamin E
- Vitamin C
- Flavonoids
- CoQ10
- Ginkgo biloba
- Alpha-lipoic acid (600 mg/day)

According to:
2. Ginkgo Biloba for Mild Cognitive Impairment and Alzheimer's Disease: A Systematic Review and Meta-Analysis of Randomized Controlled Trials. Yang G, Wang Y, Sun J, Zhang K, et al. Curr Top Med Chem. 2016;16(5):520-8. PMID: 26268332

"Ginkgo biloba is a natural medicine used for cognitive impairment and Alzheimer's disease.

"21 trials with 2608 patients met the inclusion criteria."

"Ginkgo biloba is potentially beneficial for the improvement of cognitive function, activities of daily living, and global clinical assessment in patients with mild cognitive impairment or Alzheimer's disease."

According to:
3. Efficacy and tolerability of a once daily formulation of Ginkgo biloba extract EGb 761® in Alzheimer's disease and vascular dementia: results from a randomised controlled trial. Ihl R, Tribanek M, Bachinskaya N; et al. Pharmacopsychiatry. 2012 Mar;45(2):41-6. Epub 2011 Nov 15. PMID: 22086747 DOI: 10.1055/s-0031-1291217

"A 24-week randomised controlled trial was conducted to assess the efficacy of a 240 mg once-daily preparation of Ginkgo biloba extract EGb 761® in 404 outpatients ≥ 50 years diagnosed with mild to moderate dementia (SKT 9-23), Alzheimer's disease (AD) or vascular dementia (VaD), with neuropsychiatric features (NPI total score ≥ 5)."

"EGb 761® improved cognitive functioning, neuropsychiatric symptoms and functional abilities in both types of dementia."

According to:
4. Ginkgo biloba extract (EGb 761) in Alzheimer's disease: is there any evidence? Ramassamy C, Longpré F, Christen Y. Curr Alzheimer Res. 2007 Jul;4(3):253-62. PMID: 17627482

"For centuries, extracts from the leaves of the Ginkgo biloba tree have been used as Chinese herbal medicine to treat a variety of health disorders."

"The standardized Ginkgo biloba extract EGb 761 was marketed in France and Germany 30 years ago for various vascular and cerebral deficits and is now classified as a food supplement in the United States."

"This review summarizes recent advancements in our understanding of the potential role of EGb 761 in the prevention of AD."

According to:
5. Meta-analysis of the efficacy and safety of Ginkgo biloba extract for the treatment of dementia. Hashiguchi M, Ohta Y, Shimizu M, et al. J Pharm Health Care Sci. 2015 Apr 10;1:14. eCollection 2015. PMID: 26819725 PMCID: PMC4729005 DOI: 10.1186/s40780-015-0014-7

"The aim of this study was to evaluate the efficacy and safety of Ginkgo biloba in patients with dementia in whom administration effects were reported using meta-analysis."

"Thirteen studies using the extract EGb761 met our inclusion criteria, which were duration of 12 to 52 weeks and daily dose of more than 120 mg, and included a total of 2381 patients."

"Taking a 240-mg daily dose of Ginkgo biloba extract is effective and safe in the treatment of dementia."

According to:
6. Ginkgo biloba for prevention of dementia: a systematic review and meta-analysis. Charemboon T, Jaisin K. J Med Assoc Thai. 2015 May;98(5):508-13. PMID: 26058281

"Meta-analysis of the two trials involving 5,889 participants indicated no significant difference in dementia rate between Ginkgo biloba and the placebo (347/2,951 vs. 330/2,938, odds ratio = 1.05, 95% CI 0.89-1.23) and there was no considerable heterogeneity between the trials."

"There is no convincing evidence from this review that demonstrated Ginkgo biloba in late-life can prevent the development of dementia."

According to:
7. Efficacy and adverse effects of ginkgo biloba for cognitive impairment and dementia: a systematic review and meta-analysis. Tan MS, Yu JT, Tan CC, et al. J Alzheimers Dis. 2015;43(2):589-603. PMID: 25114079 DOI: 10.3233/JAD-140837

"Research into Ginkgo biloba has been ongoing for many years, while the benefit and adverse effects of Ginkgo biloba extract EGb761 for cognitive impairment and dementia has been discussed controversially."

"Nine trials met our inclusion criteria. Trials were of 22-26 weeks duration and included 2,561 patients in total."

"In the meta-analysis, the weighted mean differences in change scores for cognition were in favor of EGb761 compared to placebo (-2.86, 95%CI -3.18; -2.54); the standardized mean differences in change scores for activities in daily living (ADLs) were also in favor of EGb761 compared to placebo (-0.36, 95%CI -0.44; -0.28); Peto OR showed a statistically significant difference from placebo for Clinicians' Global Impression of Change (CGIC) scale (1.88, 95%CI 1.54; 2.29)."

"All these benefits are mainly associated with EGb761 at a dose of 240 mg/day. For subgroup analysis in patients with neuropsychiatric symptoms, 240 mg/day EGb761 improved cognitive function, ADLs, CGIC, and also neuropsychiatric symptoms with statistical superiority than for the whole group."

"EGb761 at 240 mg/day is able to stabilize or slow decline in cognition, function, behavior, and global change at 22-26 weeks in cognitive impairment and dementia, especially for patients with neuropsychiatric symptoms."

Glutamate: ↑

The Short Story:
Defined: Glutamate is an essential amino acid and neurotransmitter naturally found in the body in a very sensitive and balanced way.

Summary: It is important to not eat foods and drinks that are processed. These contain extra flavorings (glutamate and a host of other names) which move our body's balance too high and causes overstimulation to death of our brain cells.

Lightning facts:

- A tricky balance of N-methyl-d-aspartate receptor (NMDAR) is critical for brain nervous tissue survival and excessive activity is toxic to brain cells. [1]

- "Glutamine and glutamate complex (Glx) was altered during a stimulation that may be used to evaluate **neuronal dysfunction** in a demented patient." [2]

- "Together with aspartate, glutamate is the major excitatory neurotransmitter in the brain." [3]

- "**Excess** extracellular glutamate may lead to excitotoxicity in vitro and in vivo in **acute insults** like ischemic stroke via the overactivation of ionotropic glutamate receptors." [3]
  - So neuroexcitatatory **additives** in our food and processed beverages can **overstimulate** our brain and **kill** brain cells.

The Details:

According to:

1. Role of Glutamate and NMDA Receptors in Alzheimer's Disease. Wang R, Reddy PH. J Alzheimers Dis. 2016 Sep 23. [Epub ahead of print] PMID: 27662322 DOI: 10.3233/JAD-160763

"Excitatory glutamatergic neurotransmission via N-methyl-d-aspartate receptor (NMDAR) is critical for synaptic plasticity and survival of neurons."

"However, excessive NMDAR activity causes excitotoxicity and promotes cell death, underlying a potential mechanism of neurodegeneration occurred in Alzheimer's disease (AD)."

"In contrast, the activation of extrasynaptic NMDARs promotes cell death and thus contributes to the etiology of AD, which can be blocked by an AD drug, memantine, an NMDAR antagonist that selectively blocks the function of extrasynaptic NMDARs."

According to:

2. Glutamine and Glutamate Complex, as Measured by Functional Magnetic Resonance Spectroscopy, Alters During Face-Name Association Task in Patients with Mild Cognitive Impairment and Alzheimer's Disease. Jahng GH, Oh J, Lee DW, et al. J Alzheimers Dis. 2016 Mar 5;52(1):145-59. PMID: 27060946 DOI: 10.3233/JAD-150877.

"Glutamine and glutamate complex (Glx) was statistically significantly different between the fixation and repeat conditions in aMCI (p=0.0492) as well as between the fixation and the novel conditions in the AD (p=0.0412) group."

"Glx was altered during a stimulation that may be used to evaluate neuronal dysfunction in a demented patient."

According to:
3. Chronic Glutamate Toxicity in Neurodegenerative Diseases-What is the Evidence? Lewerenz J1, Maher P2. Front Neurosci. 2015 Dec 16;9:469. eCollection 2015. PMID: 26733784 PMCID: PMC4679930 DOI: 10.3389/fnins.2015.00469

"Together with aspartate, glutamate is the major excitatory neurotransmitter in the brain."

"Although the intracellular glutamate concentration in the brain is in the millimolar range, the extracellular glutamate concentration is kept in the low micromolar range by the action of excitatory amino acid transporters that import glutamate and aspartate into astrocytes and neurons."

"Excess extracellular glutamate may lead to excitotoxicity in vitro and in vivo in acute insults like ischemic stroke via the overactivation of ionotropic glutamate receptors."

"In addition, we summarize the available experimental evidence for glutamate toxicity in animal models of neurodegenerative diseases."

Glutathione:

The Short Story:
Defined: The master antioxidant in our body and most importantly in our brain.

Summary: Glutathione helps our brain when injured and diseased. It in a sense cleans up the cob webs, and stops the harmful chemicals that can build up and destroy our sensitive nervous tissues.

Lightning facts:
- Glutathione (GST) is a **great marker** on examination with magnetic resonance spectroscopy with 87.5% accuracy for mild cognitive impairment and 91% sensitivity for Alzheimer's Disease. [2.]
- Glutathione **prevents oxidative** stress which is thought to be a significant possible pathological contribution leading to the activation of degenerating cascades inside nerve cells.
- "In general, there is an **association** between glutathione **depletion** and Parkinson's or Alzheimer's disease." [3.]
- **Inflammation** in our brain and blood makes Alzheimer's Disease **worse**. [4.]
- "**Protecting** brain endothelial cells under oxidative stress is **key** to treating cerebrovascular diseases and neurodegenerative diseases including Alzheimer's disease and Huntington's disease." [5.]

The Details:

According to:

1. Role of Glutathione-S-transferases in neurological problems. Kumar A, Dhull DK, Gupta V, et al. Expert Opin Ther Pat. 2016 Oct 27. [Epub ahead of print] PMID: 27785931 DOI: 10.1080/13543776.2017.1254192

"Role of Glutathione-S-transferases (GSTs) has been well explored in the cellular detoxification process, regulation of redox homeostasis and S-glutothionylation of target proteins like JNK, ASK1 etc."

"Oxidative stress is one of the possible pathological events that contributes significantly to activation of degenerating cascades inside neuronal cells."

"Furthermore, the authors have made significant efforts to discuss the regulation of different GST isoforms that have been associated with various pathological processes such as glioblastoma, Alzheimer's disease, Parkinson's disease, stroke and epilepsy."

According to:

2. Brain glutathione levels--a novel biomarker for mild cognitive impairment and Alzheimer's disease. Mandal PK, Saharan S, Tripathi M, et al. Biol Psychiatry. 2015 Nov 15;78(10):702-10. Epub 2015 Apr 14.

"In this study, we investigated GSH modulation in the brain with AD and assessed the diagnostic potential of GSH estimation in hippocampi (HP) and frontal cortices (FC) as a biomarker for AD and its prodromal stage, mild cognitive impairment (MCI)."

"Receiver operator characteristics analyses evidenced that hippocampal GSH robustly discriminates between MCI and healthy controls with 87.5% sensitivity, 100% specificity, and positive and negative likelihood ratios of 8.76/.13, whereas cortical GSH differentiates MCI and AD with 91.7% sensitivity, 100% specificity, and positive and negative likelihood ratios of 9.17/.08."

"The present study provides compelling in vivo evidence that estimation of GSH levels in specific brain regions with magnetic resonance spectroscopy constitutes a clinically relevant biomarker for MCI and AD."

According to:
3. Glutathione transferases and neurodegenerative diseases. Mazzetti AP, Fiorile MC, Primavera A, et al. Neurochem Int. 2015 Mar;82:10-8. doi: 10.1016/j.neuint.2015.01.008. Epub 2015 Feb 7. PMID: 25661512 DOI: 10.1016/j.neuint.2015.01.008

"There is substantial agreement that the unbalance between oxidant and antioxidant species may affect the onset and/or the course of a number of common diseases including Parkinson's and Alzheimer's diseases."

"In general, there is an association between glutathione depletion and Parkinson's or Alzheimer's disease."

According to:
4. Mild systemic oxidative stress in the subclinical stage of Alzheimer's disease. Giavarotti L, Simon KA, Azzalis LA, et al. Oxid Med Cell Longev. 2013;2013:609019. doi: 10.1155/2013/609019. Epub 2013 Dec 18. PMID: 24454987 PMCID: PMC3880752 DOI: 10.1155/2013/609019

"Alzheimer's disease (AD) is a late-onset, progressive degenerative disorder that affects mainly the judgment, emotional stability, and memory domains."

"We evaluated erythrocyte activities of superoxide dismutase, catalase, and glutathione peroxidase as well as plasma levels of total glutathione, α-tocopherol, β-carotene, lycopene, and coenzyme Q10."

"These findings support the inflammatory theory of AD and point out that this disease is associated with a higher basal activation of circulating monocytes that may be a result of α-tocopherol stock depletion."

According to:
5. Glutathione protects brain endothelial cells from hydrogen peroxide-induced oxidative stress by increasing nrf2 expression. Song J, Kang SM, Lee WT, et al. Exp Neurobiol. 2014 Mar;23(1):93-103. Epub 2014 Mar 27. PMID: 24737944 PMCID: PMC3984961 DOI: 10.5607/en.2014.23.1.93

"Glutathione (GSH) protects cells against oxidative stress by playing an antioxidant role. Protecting brain endothelial cells under oxidative stress is key to treating cerebrovascular diseases and neurodegenerative diseases including Alzheimer's disease and Huntington's disease."

"In present study, we investigated the protective effect of GSH on brain endothelial cells against hydrogen peroxide (H_2O_2). We showed that GSH attenuates H_2O_2-induced production of nitric oxide (NO), reactive oxygen species (ROS), and 8-Oxo-2'-deoxyguanosine (8-OHdG), an oxidized form of deoxiguanosine."

"Thus, GSH is a promising target to protect brain endothelial cells in conditions of brain injury and disease."

Eat foods rich in sources that build Glutathione:
- Avocado
- Asparagus
- Broccoli
- Garlic
- Raw Eggs
- Spinach
- Tomatoes
- Curcumin (Turmeric)

Glyphosate / Round up: ↑

The Short Story:
Defined: An artificial chemical compound that is a is a broad herbicide, particularly effective against weeds that come back each year.

Summary: Keep away from any foods that could have been grown in, near, or around glycoside herbicide.

Lightning facts:
- "Glyphosate **reduces** the number of these types of **beneficial gut bacteria**, thereby enhancing the poor absorption of these vital minerals." [1.]
- "**Zinc deficiency** along with **excess** exposure to **copper** may be a key factor in Alzheimer's disease." [1.]
- Roundup(®)-Ready feed and/or Glyphosate **severely deplete Manganese** (Mn) levels in plants and animals. [2.]
- Mn is part of a reaction to **protect** cells from damage that can result in Alzheimer's.

The Details:
According to:

1. Glyphosate's Suppression of Cytochrome P450 Enzymes and Amino Acid Biosynthesis by the Gut Microbiome: Pathways to Modern Diseases. Anthony Samsel and Stephanie Seneff, from the Massachusetts Institute of Technology (MIT). Entropy April 18, 2013, 15, pp. 1416-1463

"Glyphosate, the active ingredient in Roundup®, is the most popular herbicide used worldwide,"

"Glyphosate residues are found in the main foods of the Western diet, especially sugar, corn, soy and wheat."

"Glyphosate is toxic because it inhibits the cytochrome P450 (CYP) enzymes." These enzymes break down xenobiotics which we do not want in our body, thus lower enzymes, higher xenobiotics.

"80% of genetically modified crops, particularly corn, soy, canola, cotton, sugar beets and most recently alfalfa, are specifically targeted towards the introduction of genes resistant to glyphosate." A.k.a. Roundup Ready® crops

Glyphosate's mechanism of action is the disruption of the pathway involved in the synthesis of the essential aromatic amino acids, a pathway that is absent in all animals known as the shikimate pathway.

"However, this pathway is present in gut bacteria, which play an important and heretofore largely overlooked role in human physiology."

"Glyphosate wipes out the gut bacteria that produce tryptophan. Tryptophan is an essential amino acid. Tryptophan depletion leads to serotonin and melatonin depletion in the brain. Serotonin is a potent appetite suppressant. Serotonin deficiency leads to overeating and obesity."

"Reduced melatonin will also lead to sleep disorders."

"Glyphosate reduces the number of these types of beneficial gut bacteria, thereby enhancing the poor absorption of these vital minerals."

"Zinc deficiency along with excess exposure to copper may be a key factor in Alzheimer's disease."
"Tyrosine is synthesized from phenylalanine. Dopamine is synthesized from tyrosine. Both tyrosine and phenylalanine are depleted by glyphosate in both plants and microbes, reducing their bioavailability in the diet, reducing dopamine concentrations in the brain. Impaired dopamine signaling is a key feature of Parkinson's disease."

"Roundup® interferes with testosterone synthesis at very low concentrations."

"Glyphosate may be the most significant environmental toxin contributing to autism."

"The key pathological biological effects of glyphosate: disruption of the gut bacteria, impairment of sulfate transport, and interference with CYP enzyme activity—can easily explain the features that are characteristic of autism."

According to:

2. Glyphosate, pathways to modern diseases III: Manganese, neurological diseases, and associated pathologies. Samsel A, Seneff S. Surg Neurol Int. 2015 Mar 24;6:45.eCollection 2015. PMID: 25883837 PMCID: PMC4392553 DOI: 10.4103/2152-7806.153876

"A recent study on cows fed genetically modified Roundup(®)-Ready feed revealed a severe depletion of serum Mn. Glyphosate, the active ingredient in Roundup(®), has also been shown to severely deplete Mn levels in plants."

"Here, we investigate the impact of Mn on physiology, and its association with gut dysbiosis as well as neuropathologies such as autism, Alzheimer's disease (AD), depression, anxiety syndrome, Parkinson's disease (PD), and prion diseases."

"Mn superoxide dismutase protects mitochondria from oxidative damage, and mitochondrial dysfunction is a key feature of autism and Alzheimer's."

Iron: ↑

The Short Story:
Defined: An element of the earth essential in cellular metabolism.

Summary: As we age, it would be good to keep iron on the low side of normal when reviewing your blood labs. For gosh sakes make sure any pills / supplements you are taking **doesn't** have iron or copper!

Lightning facts:
- "**Excessive** accumulation of **iron** in subcortical and deep gray matter has been related to dementia." [1.]
- Iron may be a marker of vascular dementia and be part of its cause. [2.]
- As we age, **we want lower copper and iron** to keep our brains sharp. [3.]
- Iron **accumulation** occurs in aging causing neuronal iron levels to further **increase** in AD. [4.]
- "… excess iron is a potent source of oxidative damage through radical formation…" [5.]
- "However, an **increased** level of brain iron may promote **neurotoxicity** due to free radical formation, lipid peroxidation, and ultimately, cellular **death**." [6.]

The Details:

According to:

1. Patterns of Brain Iron Accumulation in Vascular Dementia and Alzheimer's Dementia Using Quantitative Susceptibility Mapping Imaging. Moon Y, Han SH, Moon WJ. J Alzheimers Dis. 2016;51(3):737-45. PMID: 26890777 DOI: 10.3233/JAD-151037

"Emerging evidence suggests that the excessive accumulation of iron in subcortical and deep gray matter has been related to dementia. However, the presence and pattern of iron accumulation in vascular dementia (VaD) and Alzheimer's disease (AD) are rarely investigated."

"In VaD and AD, overall susceptibility values were higher than those of control subjects. A significant difference in susceptibility values was found in the putamen and caudate nucleus (p< 0.001 and p=0.002, respectively)."

"Increased iron deposition in the putamen and caudate nucleus in VaD and AD patients was not associated with age or the severity of cognitive deficits."

According to:

2. Characterizing brain iron deposition in subcortical ischemic vascular dementia using susceptibility-weighted imaging: An in vivo MR study. Liu C, Li C, Yang J, et al. Behav Brain Res. 2015 Jul 15;288:33-8. Epub 2015 Apr 9. PMID: 25862942 DOI: 10.1016/j.bbr.2015.04.003

"The aim of this study was to investigate the brain iron accumulation in subcortical ischemic vascular dementia (SIVD) and its correlation with the severity of cognitive impairment."

"Our results suggest that brain iron deposition may be a biomarker of SIVD and play an important role in the pathophysiological mechanism."

According to:
3. Age-associated changes of brain copper, iron, and zinc in Alzheimer's disease and dementia with Lewy bodies. Graham SF, Nasaruddin MB, Carey M, et al. J Alzheimers Dis. 2014;42(4):1407-13. PMID: 25024342 DOI: 10.3233/JAD-140684

"Disease-, age-, and gender-associated changes in brain copper, iron, and zinc were assessed in postmortem neocortical tissue (Brodmann area 7) from patients with moderate Alzheimer's disease (AD) (n = 14), severe AD (n = 28), dementia with Lewy bodies (n = 15), and normal age-matched control subjects (n = 26)."

"Copper was lower (20%; $p < 0.001$) and iron higher (10-16%; $p < 0.001$) in severe AD compared with controls."

"Intriguingly significant Group*Age interactions were observed for both copper and iron, suggesting gradual age-associated decline of these metals in healthy non-cognitively impaired individuals."

According to:
4. Nucleic acid oxidative damage in Alzheimer's disease-explained by the hepcidin-ferroportin neuronal iron overload hypothesis? Hofer T, Perry G. J Trace Elem Med Biol. 2016 Dec;38:1-9. Epub 2016 Jun 7. PMID: 27329321 DOI: 10.1016/j.jtemb.2016.06.005

167

"There is strong literature support for brain metal dysregulation, oxidative stress and oxidative damage to neurons in Alzheimer's disease (AD); these processes begin early and continue throughout the disease."

"Whereas neuronal iron accumulation occurs in aging, neuronal iron levels further increase in AD accompanied by oxidative damage, decreased copper levels, amyloid plaque formation and brain inflammation."

"The 'hepcidin-ferroportin iron overload' AD hypothesis links these processes together and is discussed here."

According to:
5. Iron neurochemistry in Alzheimer's disease and Parkinson's disease: targets for therapeutics. Belaidi AA, Bush AI. J Neurochem. 2016 Oct;139 Suppl 1:179-197. Epub 2016 Feb 10. PMID: 26545340 DOI: 10.1111/jnc.13425

"Dysregulation of iron metabolism associated with cellular damage and oxidative stress is reported as a common event in several neurodegenerative disorders such as Alzheimer's, Parkinson's, and Huntington's diseases."

"Indeed, many proteins initially characterized in those diseases such as amyloid-β protein, α-synuclein, and huntingtin have been linked to iron neurochemistry."

"However, excess iron is a potent source of oxidative damage through radical formation and because of the lack of a body-wide export system, a tight regulation of its uptake, transport and storage is crucial in fulfilling cellular functions while keeping its level below the toxicity threshold."

"Iron plays a fundamental role in maintaining the high metabolic and energetic requirements of the brain."

According to:
6. Role of iron in neurotoxicity: a cause for concern in the elderly? Stankiewicz JM1, Brass SD.Curr Opin Clin Nutr Metab Care. 2009 Jan;12(1):22-9. PMID: 19057183 doi: 10.1097/MCO.0b013e32831ba07c.

"Because iron plays a role in oxygen transportation, myelin synthesis, neurotransmitter production, and electron transfers, it serves as a crucial cofactor in normal central nervous metabolism."

"However, an increased level of brain iron may promote neurotoxicity due to free radical formation, lipid peroxidation, and ultimately, cellular death."

"Advanced neuroimaging techniques and pathological studies have demonstrated increased brain iron with aging, and increased iron deposition has also been observed in patients with a constellation of neurological diseases, including Alzheimer's disease, Parkinson's disease, and stroke."

Lewy Bodies: ↑

The Short Story:
Defined: Lewy body dementia is the 2nd most common type of progressive dementia. Lewy bodies are deposits of proteins inside nerve cells interfering with memory, movement and thought.

Summary: Dementia with Lewy Bodies have significant complications vs dementia and Alzheimer's Disease.

Lightning facts:
- "Dementia with Lewy Bodies (DLB) were found to perform **significantly worse** on some measures of **attention** and **visuospatial** functioning in comparison with early AD" [1]
- "… DLB patients have relatively mild memory disturbance, fluctuating cognition; more **severe disturbances** of **attention**, **executive function**, visuospacial function, **visual hallucination**, **depression**, autonomic symptoms, **REM sleep** behavior disorder, and idiopathic parkinsonism compared to AD patients." [3]

The Details:
According to:
1. Comparing Cognitive Profiles of Licensed Drivers with Mild Alzheimer's Disease and Mild Dementia with Lewy Bodies. Yamin S, Stinchcombe A, Gagnon S. Int J Alzheimers Dis. 2016;2016:6542962. Epub 2016 Sep 27. PMID: 27774333 DOI: 10.1155/2016/6542962

"Purpose. Alzheimer's disease (AD) and dementia with Lewy Bodies (DLB) constitute two of the most common forms of dementia in North America."

"The purpose of this paper is to describe the cognitive profile of licensed drivers with mild AD and mild DLB."

"Participants with early DLB were found to perform significantly worse on some measures of attention and visuospatial functioning in comparison with early AD."

According to:
2. Metals in Alzheimer's and Parkinson's Disease: Relevance to Dementia with Lewy Bodies. McAllum EJ, Finkelstein DI. J Mol Neurosci. 2016 Nov;60(3):279-288. Epub 2016 Aug 8. PMID: 27498879 DOI: 10.1007/s12031-016-0809-5

"Despite being a common form of dementia, dementia with Lewy bodies is relatively under-researched when compared with Parkinson's disease and Alzheimer's disease."

"This review will discuss the role of biological metals in Parkinson's disease and Alzheimer's disease and whether there are indications that metals may also be involved in dementia with Lewy bodies."

According to:
3. [Dementia with Lewy bodies]. [Article in Japanese] Orimo S. Nihon Rinsho. 2016 Mar;74(3):483-8. PMID: 27025091

"It is important to differentiate dementia with Lewy bodies (DLB) and other dementia, especially Alzheimer disease (AD), because the medical treatment, management, and the prognosis of these diseases are different."

"In regard to clinical features, DLB patients have relatively mild memory disturbance, fluctuating cognition, more severe disturbances of attention, executive function, visuospacial function, visual hallucination, depression, autonomic symptoms, REM sleep behavior disorder, and idiopathic parkinsonism compared to AD patients."

"In regard to imaging tools, DLB patients have milder atrophy of medial temporal lobe by brain MRI, reduced occipital activity by SPECT or PET, reduced MIBG uptake by MIBG cardiac scintigraphy, and low dopamine transporter activity in the basal ganglia by SPECT or PET."

Lipids: ↑

The Short Story:

Defined: Organic molecules like fats, glycerides, fat soluble vitamins, and more which are important in health and functions of every cell when not oxidized / degenerated.

Summary: Make sure you take omega 3 fatty acids / fish oils to protect your body against the degeneration of the omega-6 fatty acids which can increase the risk of dementia. That combined with mid-life increase of LDL will compound that danger!

Lightning facts:

- Good news: LDL and VLDL can't carry cholesterol into the brain for help and repair, just **HDL** can cross the barrier which **protects** the brain! [1.]
- **Elevated Homocysteine** and **decreased** vitamin **A&E increase** dementia. [2.]
- "**Elevated** low-density lipoprotein (**LDL**) concentration in **mid-life increases** the risk of developing Alzheimer's disease (AD) in later life." [3.]
- **Highly processed foods** (rich in omega-6) when oxidized / broken down **increase** plaques in the brain and **progress** Alzheimer's Disease. [4.]
- "**Omega 3 Fatty Acids**, ω-3 PUFAs appear to contribute to **preventing** and **treating** AD." [4.]

The Details:

According to:

1. Linking lipids to Alzheimer's disease: cholesterol and beyond. Gilbert Di Paolo & Tae-Wan Kim Nature Reviews Neuroscience 12, 284-296 (May 2011) doi:10.1038/nrn3012

"In addition, dysregulation of lipid pathways has been implicated in a growing number of neurodegenerative disorders, such as Alzheimer's disease (AD)."

"Cholesterol in the brain is mainly derived from de novo synthesis from the endoplasmic reticulum (ER). Small amounts of cholesterol can also be delivered to the brain from the periphery through high density liproproteins (HDLs), which can cross the blood–brain barrier (BBB), whereas larger lipoproteins such as low-density lipoproteins and very low density lipoproteins (LDL/VLDL) are unable to do so (shown by the red cross)."

"Excess free cholesterol is converted into cholesterol ester by sterol O-acyltransferase 2 (ACAT; also known as acyl CoA:cholesterol acyltransferase 1)."

According to:

2. Homocysteine, antioxidant vitamins and lipids as biomarkers of neurodegeneration in Alzheimer's disease versus non-Alzheimer's dementia. Raszewski G, Chwedorowicz R, Chwedorowicz A, et al. Ann Agric Environ Med. 2016;23(1):193-6. PMID: 27007541 DOI: 10.5604/12321966.1196878

"Cognitive function was assessed by Mini-Mental State Examination (MMSE) and related to plasma levels of tHcy, folate, vitamins B-6, B-12, lipids and vitamins A and E for both groups."

"A significant reduction in serum vitamin A levels and elevation of total cholesterol levels were shown for the Dementia Patient (DP-s) group compared to those in the control group."

"The results obtained suggest that elevated serum tHcy and decreased levels of vitamins A and E are associated with an increased risk of non-Alzheimer's dementias, although further studies involving a larger cohort are now needed to verify these results."

According to:
3. LDL-lipids from patients with hypercholesterolaemia and Alzheimer's disease are inflammatory to microvascular endothelial cells: mitigation by statin intervention.
Dias HK, Brown CL, Polidori MC, et al. Clin Sci (Lond). 2015 Dec;129(12):1195-206. Epub 2015 Sep 23. PMID: 26399707 PMCID: PMC5055810 DOI: 10.1042/CS20150351

"Elevated low-density lipoprotein (LDL) concentration in mid-life increases the risk of developing Alzheimer's disease (AD) in later life."

"Only hyperlipidaemic subjects with normal cognitive function received 40 mg of simvastatin intervention/day for 3 months."

"LDL-L isolated after statin intervention did not affect endothelial function. In summary, LDL-L from hypercholesterolaemic, AD and AD-plus patients are inflammatory to (Human microvascular endothelial cells) HMVECs. In vivo intervention with statins reduces the damaging effects of LDL-L on HMVECs."

According to:
4. Dietary lipids and their oxidized products in Alzheimer's disease. Corsinovi L, Biasi F, Poli G, et al. Mol Nutr Food Res. 2011 Sep;55 Suppl 2:S161-72. Epub 2011 Aug 31. PMID: 21954186 DOI: 10.1002/mnfr.201100208

"A growing body of scientific literature addresses the implication of dietary habits in the pathogenesis of AD."

"Oxidative breakdown products of ω-6 polyunsaturated fatty acids (ω-6 PUFAs), and cholesterol oxidation products (oxysterols), might play a role in favoring β-amyloid deposition, a hallmark of AD's onset and progression."

"Conversely, ω-3 PUFAs appear to contribute to preventing and treating AD."

"The use of a diet with an appropriate ω-3/ω-6 PUFA ratio, rich in healthy oils, fish and antioxidants, such as flavonoids, but low in cholesterol-containing foods, can be a beneficial component in the clinical strategies of prevention of AD."

According to:
5. Association of blood lipids with Alzheimer's disease: A comprehensive lipidomics analysis. Proitsi P, Kim M, Whiley L, et al. Alzheimers Dement. 2016 Sep 28. pii: S1552-5260(16)30022-X. PMID: 27693183 DOI: 10.1016/j.jalz.2016.08.003

"The aim of this study was to (1) replicate previous associations between six blood lipids and Alzheimer's disease (AD) (Proitsi et al 2015) and (2) identify novel associations between lipids, clinical AD diagnosis, disease progression and brain atrophy (left/right hippocampus/entorhinal cortex)."

"We putatively identified a number of metabolic features including cholesteryl esters/triglycerides and phosphatidylcholines."

Magnesium: ↓

The Short Story:
Defined: Magnesium is the fourth most abundant mineral in the body.

Summary: Either eat foods rich in magnesium or take a quality supplement to make sure your magnesium levels do not get low.

Lightning facts:
- "**Low** levels of **magnesium** have been associated with a number of chronic diseases, such as **Alzheimer's** disease, insulin resistance and type-2 diabetes mellitus, hypertension, cardiovascular disease (e.g., stroke), migraine headaches, and attention deficit hyperactivity disorder (ADHD)." [1.]
- AD seems to be associated with a lower Mg status when compared to healthy controls." [2.]
- "**Iron**-induced fibrin fibers can **irreversibly** trap red blood cells (RBCs) and in this way obstruct oxygen delivery to the brain and **induce chronic hypoxia** that may contribute to AD." [3.]
- "The RBC-fibrin aggregates can be **disaggregated** by **magnesium** ions and can also be **prevented** by certain polyphenols that are known to have beneficial effects in AD." [3.]
- "Our data suggest that there is a relationship between serum Mg levels and the degree of Alzheimer's disease." [4.]

The Details:

According to:

1. Magnesium in Prevention and Therapy. Gröber U, Schmidt J, Kisters K. Nutrients. 2015 Sep 23;7(9):8199-226. PMID: 26404370 PMCID: PMC4586582 DOI: 10.3390/nu7095388

"It has been recognized as a cofactor for more than 300 enzymatic reactions, where it is crucial for adenosine triphosphate (ATP) metabolism. Magnesium is required for DNA and RNA synthesis, reproduction, and protein synthesis."

"Moreover, magnesium is essential for the regulation of muscular contraction, blood pressure, insulin metabolism, cardiac excitability, vasomotor tone, nerve transmission and neuromuscular conduction."

"Low levels of magnesium have been associated with a number of chronic diseases, such as Alzheimer's disease, insulin resistance and type-2 diabetes mellitus, hypertension, cardiovascular disease (e.g., stroke), migraine headaches, and attention deficit hyperactivity disorder (ADHD)."

According to:

2. Magnesium Status in Alzheimer's Disease: A Systematic Review. Veronese N, Zurlo A, Solmi M, et al. Am J Alzheimers Dis Other Demen. 2016 May;31(3):208-13. Epub 2015 Sep 7. PMID: 26351088 DOI: 10.1177/1533317515602674

"The interest in poor magnesium (Mg) status as risk factor for Alzheimer's disease (AD) is increasing due to its antioxidant and neuroprotective properties."

"Of 192 potentially eligible studies, 13 were included (559 patients with AD, 381 HCs, and 126 MCs)."

"In conclusion, AD seems to be associated with a lower Mg status when compared to healthy controls (HCs), while the scarcity of studies limited the findings about medical controls/illnesses (MCs)."

According to:
3. The role of iron-induced fibrin in the pathogenesis of Alzheimer's disease and the protective role of magnesium. Lipinski B, Pretorius E. Front Hum Neurosci. 2013 Oct 29;7:735. PMID: 24194714 PMCID: PMC3810650 DOI: 10.3389/fnhum.2013.00735

"One such component is fibrin clots, which, when they become resistant to thrombolysis, can cause chronic inflammation."

"This phenomenon can now be explained in terms of the iron-induced free radicals that generate fibrin-like polymers remarkably resistant to the proteolytic degradation."

"In addition, iron-induced fibrin fibers can irreversibly trap red blood cells (RBCs) and in this way obstruct oxygen delivery to the brain and induce chronic hypoxia that may contribute to AD."

"The RBC-fibrin aggregates can be disaggregated by magnesium ions and can also be prevented by certain polyphenols that are known to have beneficial effects in AD."

"In conclusion, we argue that AD can be prevented by: (1) limiting the dietary supply of trivalent iron contained in red and processed meat; (2) increasing the intake of chlorophyll-derived magnesium; and (3) consumption of foods rich in polyphenolic substances and certain aliphatic and aromatic unsaturated compounds."

According to:
4. Serum magnesium level and clinical deterioration in Alzheimer's disease. Cilliler AE, Ozturk S, Ozbakir S. Gerontology. 2007;53(6):419-22. Epub 2007 Nov 8. PMID: 17992016 DOI: 10.1159/000110873

"Recent studies suggest that magnesium, which specially affects the N-methyl-D-aspartate receptor response to excitatory amino acids, may be a supportive therapeutic agent in Alzheimer's disease."

"Our data suggest that there is a relationship between serum Mg levels and the degree of Alzheimer's disease and that the determination of the Mg level at various stages may provide valuable information in further understanding the progression and treatment of Alzheimer's disease."

Medications: ↑

The Short Story:
Defined: Certain drugs prescribed for conditions can have side effects, in this case, **increased** risk of dementia and Alzheimer's Disease.

Summary: Take drugs cautiously and with the least frequency possible. When all possible, look for **alternative** ways to treat the condition and make sure you know if the drugs you are taking **increase** your risk.

Lightning facts:
- In order to keep the book less than 500 pages, I would refer you to the Aging Brain Care. They have an anticholinergic cognitive burden scale 2012 update, there are **over 60 medications** listed, for example: [1,3]
  - **Sleep aids:** example: Wellbutrin
  - **Reflux** problems: example: Zyrtec , Nexium, Prevacid and Prilosec.
  - **Blood Presure** problems: example: Lasix
  - **Depression** problems: example: Effexor
  - **Allergy** problems: example: Benadryl
- **Each** definite anticholinergic may **increase** the risk of cognitive impairment by **46%** over 6 years. [2]
- "Long-term use of the drugs significantly increased the risk of developing dementia, including Alzheimer's disease." [4]

- "Though you may have never heard of this class of drug, you've certainly heard of the medications themselves, including **Benadryl**, Demerol, **Dimetapp**, Dramamine, Paxil, Unisom and VESIcare. They are sold over the counter and by prescription as sleep aids and for chronic diseases including **hypertension**, cardiovascular disease and chronic obstructive pulmonary disease (**COPD**)." [5]

The Details:
According to:
1. For further information please go to: www.agingbraincare.org.

According to:
2. JAMA NeurologyOriginal InvestigationApril 1, 2016 Association of Proton Pump Inhibitors With Risk of Dementia: A Pharmacoepidemiological Claims Data Analysis. Willy Gomm, PhD; Klaus von Holt, MD, PhD; Friederike Thomé, MSc; et al. JAMA Neurol. 2016; 73(4):410-416. doi: 10.1001/jamaneurol.2015.4791a

"Heartburn medications may be linked to a higher risk of dementia, according to a recent study."

"A total of 73 679 participants 75 years of age or older and free of dementia at baseline were analyzed. The patients receiving regular PPI medication (n = 2950; mean [SD] age, 83.8 [5.4] years; 77.9% female) had a significantly increased risk of incident dementia compared with the patients not receiving PPI medication (n = 70 729; mean [SD] age, 83.0 [5.6] years; 73.6% female) (hazard ratio, 1.44 [95% CI, 1.36-1.52]; P < .001)."

"So far, they have found a potential increased risk via the brands Nexium, Prevacid and Prilosec, with findings showing that people 75 and older who regularly take PPIs had a 44 percent increased risk of dementia when compared to seniors not taking the drugs."

According to:
3. Common Meds Linked to Dementia By Peter Russell WebMD Health News Reviewed by Hansa D. Bhargava, MD April 20, 2016

"Older people who take certain medicines to treat conditions like urinary incontinence, depression, asthma, allergies, and sleeping problems should be warned that their use may bring a higher risk of dementia, scientists say."

"The researchers say that although a link has been found before, this might be the first time that their effect at blocking a brain chemical called acetylcholine has been implicated."

"Tests on their brain function revealed that those taking the anticholinergic medications did worse than those not taking the drugs. These included results on short-term memory, verbal reasoning, planning, and problem solving."

"Another discovery was that volunteers using anticholinergic drugs had less brain volume and larger ventricles, the cavities inside the brain."

According to:
4. ALZinfo.org, The Alzheimer's Information Site. Reviewed by William J. Netzer, Ph.D., Fisher Center for Alzheimer's Research Foundation at The Rockefeller University. Source: Shelly L. Gray, PharmD, MS; Melissa L. Anderson, MS; Sascha Dublin, MD, PhD, et al: "Cumulative Use of Strong Anticholinergic Medications and Incident Dementia: A Prospective Cohort Study." JAMA Internal Medicine, January 26, 2015
https://www.alzinfo.org/articles/treatment/common-allergy-and-sleep-drugs-tied-to-higher-alzheimers-risk/

"And the longer the medications are taken, the greater the risk."

"The drugs include many popular prescription and over-the-counter medications. They include tricyclic antidepressants like doxepin (Sinequan), antihistamines like chlorpheniramine (Chlor-Trimeton) and diphenhydramine (Benadryl), and bladder control drugs like oxybutynin (Ditropan)."

"All of the medications are known to block a brain chemical called acetylcholine, which transmits nerve signals throughout the brain and nervous system."

""Older adults should be aware that many medications — including some available without a prescription, such as over-the-counter sleep aids — have strong anticholinergic effects," said study author Shelly Gray, director of the geriatric pharmacy program at the University of Washington School of Pharmacy."

"A link between sleep aids and dementia had been reported in earlier studies."

"The study is also the first to suggest that adverse effects of using such drugs may persist long after people stop using them, and may not be reversible. The findings appeared in JAMA Internal Medicine, from the American Medical Association."

"The researchers found that over all, long-term use of the drugs significantly increased the risk of developing dementia, including Alzheimer's disease. The study found, for example, that people taking at least 10 milligrams per day of doxepin (Sinequan, a sleep and depression aid), 4 milligrams a day of diphenhydramine (Benadryl, for allergies or sleep), or 5 milligrams a day of oxybutynin (a bladder control drug) for more than three years would be at increased risk for developing dementia."

"Instead, Dr. Gray said, patients might substitute other drugs that do not have anticholinergic effects, such as a selective serotonin re-uptake inhibitor (SSRI) like citalopram (Celexa) or fluoxitene (Prozac) for depression and a second-generation antihistamine like loratadine (Claritin) for allergies."

Mercury: ↑

The Short Story:
Defined: The Atomic Number of this element is 80 and the Element Symbol is Hg.

Summary: Mercury is toxic to you and your nervous system. Even fillings in your teeth can **increase** your Alzheimer's risk!

Lightning facts:
- An average adult should **limit to 200g of fish per week** to limit mercury exposure allowed in fish. [1.]
- The US limit of mercury allowed in the fish we consume is 250% higher than Japan's limit.   [1.]
- "Farmed finfish and shellfish that are fed fish-meal, however, can bioconcentrate both MeHg (in muscle) and organohalogen pollutants passed on in the fat components" [2.]
- **Fillings** from mercury (aka amalgam) increased risk of dementia and Alzheimer's: [3.]
  - **Women increased 13.2%**
  - **Men increased 7%**
- From a **summary of 106 studies**, mercury binds with selenium and therefore may promote nervous system disorders: dementia, Alzheimer's Disease …. [4.]

The Details:

According to:

1. Adverse Effects of Methylmercury: Environmental Health Research Implications. Philippe Grandjean, Hiroshi Satoh, Katsuyuki Murata, et al. Department of Environmental Medicine, University of Southern Denmark, Odense, Denmark; Department of Environmental Health, Harvard School of Public Health, Boston, Massachusetts, USA; Department of Environmental Health Sciences, Tohoku University Graduate School of Medicine, Sendai, Japan; Division of Environmental Health Sciences, Akita University, Akita, Japan; National Institute for Minamata Disease, Minamata, Japan Environ Health Perspect 118:1137-1145 (2010). http://dx.doi.org/10.1289/ehp.0901757 [online 01 August 2010]

"A total weekly seafood intake including two fish dinners would represent about 500 g of seafood."

However, current regulations in the United States and the European Union allow up to 10 times as much than the suggested upper limit by the EPA. By this safe limit, no more than 200g of fish per week for an average 70kg adult.

A provisionally tolerable limit of 0.4 µg/g (as total mercury, and 0.3 µg/g as methylmercury) was set by the Japanese Ministry of Health and Welfare for fish intended for human consumption (Endo et al. 2005).

According to:
2. Studies of fish consumption as source of methylmercury should consider fish-meal-fed farmed fish and other animal foods. Dórea JG. Environ Res. 2009 Jan;109(1):131-2; discussion 133-4. doi: 10.1016/j.envres.2008.10.004. Epub 2008 Nov 21. PMID: 19027108 [PubMed - indexed for MEDLINE]

"The co-occurrence of fish MeHg and omega-3 fatty acids in wild species can indeed be optimized by choosing certain species."

"Farmed finfish and shellfish that are fed fish-meal, however, can bioconcentrate both MeHg (in muscle) and organohalogen pollutants passed on in the fat components [Dorea, J.G., 2006]. Fish meal in animal feed and human exposure to persistent bioaccumulative and toxic substances. J. Food Prot. 69, 2777-2785]"

According to:
3. Association between dental amalgam fillings and Alzheimer's disease: a population-based cross-sectional study in Taiwan. Sun YH, Nfor ON, Huang JY,et al. Alzheimers Res Ther. 2015 Nov 12;7(1):65. PMID: 26560125 PMCID: PMC4642684 DOI: 10.1186/s13195-015-0150-1

"The aim of the study was to evaluate the association between dental amalgam fillings and Alzheimer's disease in Taiwanese population aged 65 and older."

"Data were retrieved from the Longitudinal Health Insurance Database (LHID 2005 and 2010). The study enrolled 1,943,702 beneficiaries from the LHID database."

"Individuals exposed to amalgam fillings had higher risk of Alzheimer's disease (odds ratio, OR = 1.105, 95 % confidence interval, CI = 1.025-1.190) than their non-exposed counterparts. Further analysis showed that the odds ratio of Ahlzheimer's disease was 1.07 (95 % CI = 0.962-1.196) in men and 1.132 (95 % CI = 1.022-1.254) in women."

"Women who were exposed to amalgam fillings were 1.132 times more likely to have Alzheimer's disease than were their non-exposed counterparts."

According to:
4. Does inorganic mercury play a role in Alzheimer's disease? A systematic review and an integrated molecular mechanism. Mutter J, Curth A, Naumann J, et al. J Alzheimers Dis. 2010;22(2):357-74. doi: 10.3233/JAD-2010-100705.

"Mercury is one of the most toxic substances known to humans. It has been introduced into the human environment and has also been widely used in medicine."

"Since circumstantial evidence exists that the pathology of Alzheimer's disease (AD) might be in part caused or exacerbated by inorganic mercury, we conducted a systematic review using a comprehensive search strategy."

"One thousand and forty-one references were scrutinized, and 106 studies fulfilled the inclusion criteria."

"Its high affinity for selenium and selenoproteins suggests that inorganic mercury may promote neurodegenerative disorders via disruption of redox regulation. Inorganic mercury may play a role as a co-factor in the development of AD."

Music: ↓

The Short Story:
Defined: The art of arranging sounds with respect to time expressing ideas and emotions through melody, harmony, rhythm, and timbre.

Summary: Music helps dementia and Alzheimer's Disease. Cheap, easy, available with no side effects!

Lightning facts:
- Music can help the **emotional** and **behavioral** status of patients. [1]
- "… analysis revealed three ways in which music influences the lives of community-dwelling older adults with **dementia**: (a) **reduced agitation**, (b) **improved cognition**, and (c) enhanced social well-being." [2]
- "Significant improvement was observed in **memory, orientation, depression** and **anxiety** (HAD scale) in **both mild and moderate** cases; in **anxiety** (NPI scale) in **mild** cases; and in **delirium, hallucinations, agitation, irritability**, and language disorders in the group with **moderate** Alzheimer disease." [3]
- "Music therapy exerted a moderately large effect on **disruptive** behaviours of people with dementia, a **moderate** effect on **anxiety** levels and **depressive** moods, and a small effect on cognitive functioning." [4]

192

- "The proposed model can be considered a low-cost nonpharmacological intervention and a therapeutic-rehabilitation method for the **reduction** of **behavioral disturbances**, for **stimulation** of **cognitive functions**, and for **increasing** the overall **quality of life** of persons with dementia." [7.]

The Details:
According to:
1. Efficacy of musical interventions in dementia: methodological requirements of nonpharmacological trials. Samson S, Clément S, Narme P, et al. Ann N Y Acad Sci. 2015 Mar;1337:249-55. PMID: 25773641 DOI: 10.1111/nyas.12621

"Consequently, the development of nondrug care, such as musical interventions, has become a necessity."

"As part of a series of studies, we carried out randomized controlled trials to compare the effectiveness of musical activities to other pleasant activities on various functions in patients with severe Alzheimer's disease."

"Although the results demonstrate the power of music on the emotional and behavioral status of patients, they also suggest that other pleasant activities (e.g., cooking) are also effective, leaving open the question about the specific benefits of music in patients with dementia."

According to:
2. The role of music in the lives of older adults with dementia ageing in place: A scoping review. Elliott M, Gardner P. Dementia (London). 2016 Mar 18. PMID: 26993049 DOI: 10.1177/1471301216639424

"Music is emerging as an effective therapeutic strategy for older adults with dementia however, most of the work to date has focused on institutions."

"Using a five-stage framework for conducting a scoping review, analysis revealed three ways in which music influences the lives of community-dwelling older adults with dementia: (a) reduced agitation, (b) improved cognition, and (c) enhanced social well-being."

According to:
3. Music therapy and Alzheimer's disease: Cognitive, psychological, and behavioural effects. Gómez Gallego M, Gómez García J. Neurologia. 2016 Feb 17. pii: S0213-4853(16)00004-9. PMID: 26896913 DOI: 10.1016/j.nrl.2015.12.003 [Article in English, Spanish]

"Music therapy is one of the types of active ageing programmes which are offered to elderly people."

The usefulness of this programme in the field of dementia is beginning to be recognised by the scientific community, since studies have reported physical, cognitive, and psychological benefits.

"Significant improvement was observed in memory, orientation, depression and anxiety (HAD scale) in both mild and moderate cases; in anxiety (NPI scale) in mild cases; and in delirium, hallucinations, agitation, irritability, and language disorders in the group with moderate Alzheimer disease."

"The effect on cognitive measures was appreciable after only 4 music therapy sessions."

"In the sample studied, music therapy improved some cognitive, psychological, and behavioural alterations in patients with Alzheimer disease."

According to:
4. The efficacy of music therapy for people with dementia: A meta-analysis of randomised controlled trials. Chang YS, Chu H, Yang CY, et al. J Clin Nurs. 2015 Dec;24(23-24):3425-40. Epub 2015 Aug 24. PMID: 26299594 DOI: 10.1111/jocn.12976

"Present study was the first to perform a meta-analysis that included all the randomised controlled trials found in literature relating to music therapy for people with dementia over the past 15 years."

"Music therapy exerted a moderately large effect on disruptive behaviours of people with dementia, a moderate effect on anxiety levels and depressive moods, and a small effect on cognitive functioning."

According to:
5. Effects of Meditation versus Music Listening on Perceived Stress, Mood, Sleep, and Quality of Life in Adults with Early Memory Loss: A Pilot Randomized Controlled Trial.
Innes KE, Selfe TK, Khalsa DS, et al. J Alzheimers Dis. 2016 Apr 8;52(4):1277-98. PMID: 27079708 DOI: 10.3233/JAD-151106

"Older adults with subjective cognitive decline (SCD) are at increased risk not only for Alzheimer's disease, but for poor mental health, impaired sleep, and diminished quality of life (QOL), which in turn, contribute to further cognitive decline, highlighting the need for early intervention."

"Observed gains were sustained or improved at 6 months, with both groups showing marked and significant improvement in all outcomes."

According to:
6. Music and Memory in Alzheimer's Disease and The Potential Underlying Mechanisms. Peck KJ, Girard TA, Russo FA, Fiocco AJ. J Alzheimers Dis. 2016;51(4):949-59. PMID: 26967216 DOI: 10.3233/JAD-150998

"A growing body of evidence suggests that music exposure can enhance memory and emotional function in persons with AD."

"Specifically, this paper will outline the potential role of the dopaminergic system, the autonomic nervous system, and the default network in explaining how music may enhance memory function in persons with AD."

According to:
7. Global music approach to persons with dementia: evidence and practice. Raglio A, Filippi S, Bellandi D,et al. Clin Interv Aging. 2014 Oct 6;9:1669-76. eCollection 2014. PMID: 25336931 PMCID: PMC4199985 DOI: 10.2147/CIA.S71388

"Music is an important resource for achieving psychological, cognitive, and social goals in the field of dementia."

"From the literature analysis the following evidence-based interventions emerged: active music therapy (psychological and rehabilitative approaches), active music therapy with family caregivers and persons with dementia, music-based interventions, caregivers singing, individualized listening to music, and background music."

"The proposed model can be considered a low-cost nonpharmacological intervention and a therapeutic-rehabilitation method for the reduction of behavioral disturbances, for stimulation of cognitive functions, and for increasing the overall quality of life of persons with dementia."

NSAIDS: ↕

The Short Story:
Defined: Non-steroidal Anti-inflammataory Drugs
(NSAids) is a medication to reduce fever, pain and
inflammation.

Summary: These medications are way too often used and
while most patients know it can cause harm to their
stomach, liver and kidneys, let's put on top the addition of
dementia and Alzheimer's.

Lightning facts:
- **Heavy** NSAID users **increased** onset of **dementia**
  by 66% and **Alzheimer's** Disease by 57%. [1.]
- It does **not prevent** Alzheimer's or dementia as
  previously thought. [1.]
- "While long-term use of NSAIDs is associated with
  a **reduced** incidence of AD in epidemiologic
  studies, randomized controlled trials have **not**
  replicated these findings." [2.]
- "Thus, NSAID use **cannot** currently be
  recommended either for primary prevention or
  treatment of AD." [2.]
- "**More** than 15 epidemiological **studies** have since
  showed a sparing effect of non-steroidal anti-
  inflammatory drugs (NSAIDs) in AD. A **consistent**
  finding has been that the **longer** the NSAIDs were
  used **prior** to clinical diagnosis, the greater the
  sparing effect." [3.]

The Details:

According to:

1. Risk of dementia and AD with prior exposure to NSAIDs in an elderly community-based cohort. Breitner JC, Haneuse SJ, Walker R, et al. Neurology. 2009 Jun 2;72(22):1899-905. Epub 2009 Apr 22. PMID: 19386997 PMCID: PMC2690966 DOI: 10.1212/WNL.0b013e3181a18691

"Nonsteroidal anti-inflammatory drugs (NSAIDs) may prevent Alzheimer dementia (AD)."

"Contrary to the hypothesis that NSAIDs protect against AD, pharmacy-defined heavy NSAID users showed increased incidence of dementia and AD, with adjusted hazard ratios of 1.66 (95% confidence interval, 1.24-2.24) and 1.57 (95% confidence interval, 1.10-2.23).

Contrary to the hypothesis that NSAIDs protect against AD, pharmacydefined heavy NSAID users showed increased incidence of dementia and AD, by 66%.

Inflammatory mechanisms are probably involved in the pathogenesis of Alzheimer dementia (AD).

"NSAIDs are not helpful for people with established AD dementia."

NSAIDs offer no benefit to people whose preclinical AD pathology is sufficiently advanced that they develop dementia symptoms within a few years.

According to:
2. Targeting neuroinflammation in Alzheimer's disease: evidence for NSAIDs and novel therapeutics. Deardorff WJ, Grossberg GT. Expert Rev Neurother. 2016 Jun 24:1-16. [Epub ahead of print]

"As immune system modulators, non-steroidal anti-inflammatory drugs (NSAIDs) garnered initial enthusiasm from pre-clinical and epidemiologic studies as agents to reduce the risk of AD."

"While long-term use of NSAIDs is associated with a reduced incidence of AD in epidemiologic studies, randomized controlled trials have not replicated these findings."

"Thus, NSAID use cannot currently be recommended either for primary prevention or treatment of AD."

According to:
3. Inflammation, Anti-inflammatory Agents, and Alzheimer's Disease: The Last 22 Years. McGeer PL, Rogers J, McGeer EG. J Alzheimers Dis. 2016 Oct 4;54(3):853-857. PMID: 27716676 DOI: 10.3233/JAD-160488

"Two basic discoveries spurred research into inflammation as a driving force in the pathogenesis of Alzheimer's disease (AD). The first was the identification of activated microglia in association with the lesions. The second was the discovery that rheumatoid arthritics, who regularly consume anti-inflammatory agents, were relatively spared from the disease."

"More than 15 epidemiological studies have since showed a sparing effect of non-steroidal anti-inflammatory drugs (NSAIDs) in AD. A consistent finding has been that the longer the NSAIDs were used prior to clinical diagnosis, the greater the sparing effect."

Obesity: ↑

The Short Story:
Defined: When a person has over 30% of the body weight in fat.

Summary: Thebest thing is to not have any more weight on you than absolutely necessary. I know it sounds logical and simple but it is EXPENSIVE if you carry weight for it will bring lifelong problems that you will have to pay to have treated totaling in the thousands and thousands of dollars, increasing in cost in the end of life. Now is the time to plan a slow weight loss process for years and decades to come vs the fad diet that leaves you fatter in 6 months to a year than when you started after you quit and go back to the habits you once had.

Lightning facts:
- Abdominal fat and being **obese** in the **waist** specifically have over **260% increase** risk in dementia!!! [1.]
  - Obese (BMI ≥ 30 kg/m2)
- Just being **overweight** with the majority of the excess in the **central** body / abdomen, increased the dementia risk 134%!! [1.]
  - Overweight (BMI = 25–29.9 kg/m2).
- **"Diabetes mellitus** (DM) type 2, **smoking**, physical **inactivity**, overweight and **obesity** were **significantly** associated with **increased** risk of AD." [2.]
- "Peripheral inflammation observed in obesity leads to insulin resistance and type 2 diabetes." [3.]

- Obese below the age of 65 **increased** dementia by 41% and has a **negative** 17% when it occurred after 65 years of age! [4.]
- Insulin resistance in children and adolescents present higher risk of developing cognitive impairment, dementia and AD. [5.]
- "Numerous studies have demonstrated that both obesity and metabolic disorders are associated with poorer cognitive performance, cognitive decline, and dementia." [6.]
- "...figures from the Organization for Economic Co-operation and Development **2014** Obesity report (OECD, 2014) suggest that **worldwide 18% of the adult population are obese**, with more than one in three adults in Mexico, New Zealand and the United States, and more than one in four in Australia, Canada, Chile, and Hungary included in this category." [6.]
- Another study says that over the relative risk of the development of dementia and Alzheimer's disease for **obese** and **overweight** individuals in midlife compared to normal weight individuals was **2.04** and **1.64**, respectively (Anstey et al., 2011). [6.]
- Fat cell dysfunction and abnormal fat production are involved in dementia since they **can cross** the blood-brain barrier and influence thought-related structures. [7.]
- Fat hormones (adipokines) made from fat tissue have vast influence in the brain and in the body! They can cross the blood brain barrier so can freely go in and out of the brain! [9.]

The Details:

According to:
1. Central obesity and increased risk of dementia more than three decades later. R.A. Whitmer, PhD; D.R. Gustafson, PhD; E. Barrett-Connor, MD; et al. Neurology; March 26, 2008.

"A longitudinal analysis was conducted of 6,583 members of Kaiser Permanente of Northern California who had their sagittal abdominal diameter (SAD) measured from 1964 to 1973."

Those both obese and with high SAD had the highest risk of dementia, with an increased risk by 260%.

"Obesity, as measured by body mass index (BMI), particularly in middle age, increases the risk of dementia, Alzheimer disease (AD), and neurodegenerative changes."

"Overweight and with central obesity had a 134% increase in dementia risk."

According to:
2. Population attributable fraction of modifiable risk factors for Alzheimer disease: A systematic review of systematic reviews. Hazar N, Seddigh L, Rampisheh Z, et al. Iran J Neurol. 2016 Jul 6;15(3):164-72. PMID: 27648178 PMCID: PMC5027152

"The aim of the current review was to characterize modifiable cardiovascular risk factors of AD using existing data and determine their contribution in AD development in Iran and the world."

"Of 2651 articles, 11 were eligible for data extraction after assessing relevancy and quality. Diabetes mellitus (DM) type 2, smoking, physical inactivity, overweight and obesity were significantly associated with increased risk of AD. Physical inactivity with 22.0% and smoking with 15.7% had the highest population attributable fraction (PAF) for AD in Iran and the world, respectively."

According to:
3. Common neurodegenerative pathways in obesity, diabetes, and Alzheimer's disease. Pugazhenthi S, Qin L, Reddy PH. Biochim Biophys Acta. 2016 May 6. pii: S0925-4439(16)30097-7. PMID: 27156888 DOI: 10.1016/j.bbadis.2016.04.017

"Studies have identified several overlapping neurodegenerative mechanisms, including oxidative stress, mitochondrial dysfunction, and inflammation that are observed in these disorders."

"Peripheral inflammation observed in obesity leads to insulin resistance and type 2 diabetes."

"Damage to the blood brain barrier (BBB) as seen with aging can lead to infiltration of immune cells into the brain, leading to the exacerbation of central inflammation."

"This review discusses these molecular mechanisms that link obesity, diabetes and AD."

According to:
4. The risk of overweight/obesity in mid-life and late life for the development of dementia: a systematic review and meta-analysis of longitudinal studies. Pedditizi E, Peters R, Beckett N. Age Ageing. 2016 Jan;45(1):14-21. PMID: 26764391 DOI: 10.1093/ageing/afv151

"Corrigenda: Corrigendum to 'The risk of overweight/obesity in mid-life and late life for the development of dementia: a systematic review and meta-analysis of longitudinal studies'. [Age Ageing. 2016]"

"Of the 1,612 abstracts identified and reviewed, 21 completely met the inclusion criteria. Being obese below the age of 65 years had a positive association on incident dementia with a risk ratio (RR) 1.41 (95% confidence interval, CI: 1.20-1.66), but the opposite was seen in those aged 65 and over, RR 0.83 (95% CI: 0.74-0.94)."

According to:
5. Biomarkers of Alzheimer disease, insulin resistance, and obesity in childhood. Luciano R, Barraco GM, Muraca M, et al. Pediatrics. 2015 Jun;135(6):1074-81. Epub 2015 May 11. PMID: 25963004 DOI: 10.1542/peds.2014-2391

"To answer the question of whether onset of insulin resistance (IR) early in life enhances the risk of developing dementia and Alzheimer disease (AD), serum levels of 2 molecules that are likely associated with development of AD, the amyloid β-protein 42 (Aβ42) and presenilin 1 (PSEN1), were estimated in 101 preschoolers and 309 adolescents of various BMI."

"Obese adolescents with IR present higher levels of circulating molecules that might be associated with increased risk of developing later in elderly cognitive impairment, dementia, and AD."

According to:
6. Obesity and cognitive decline: role of inflammation and vascular changes. Nguyen JC, Killcross AS, Jenkins TA. Front Neurosci. 2014 Nov 19;8:375. eCollection 2014. PMID: 25477778 PMCID: PMC4237034 DOI: 10.3389/fnins.2014.00375

"The incidence of obesity in middle age is increasing markedly, and in parallel the prevalence of metabolic disorders including cardiovascular disease and type II diabetes is also rising."

"Numerous studies have demonstrated that both obesity and metabolic disorders are associated with poorer cognitive performance, cognitive decline, and dementia."

"In this review we discuss the effects of obesity on cognitive performance, including both clinical and preclinical observations, and discuss some of the potential mechanisms involved, namely inflammation and vascular and metabolic alterations."

"Attributed to unhealthy diets (that is over-consumption of food and beverages with a high content of fats, sugars, and salt) and physical inactivity, figures from the Organization for Economic Co-operation and Development 2014 Obesity report (OECD, 2014) suggest that worldwide 18% of the adult population are obese, with more than one in three adults in Mexico, New Zealand and the United States, and more than one in four in Australia, Canada, Chile, and Hungary included in this category."

"Obesity is associated with not only an increased risk of development of mild cognitive impairment, but additionally, late-life dementia and Alzheimer's disease (Solfrizzi et al., 2004; Whitmer et al., 2005; Gustafson et al., 2012; Besser et al., 2014)."

"The relative risk of the development of dementia and Alzheimer's disease for obese (BMI $\geq$ 30 kg/m2) and overweight (BMI = 25–29.9 kg/m2) individuals in midlife compared to normal weight individuals was 2.04 and 1.64, respectively (Anstey et al., 2011)."

According to:
7. Obesity as a risk factor for Alzheimer's disease: the role of adipocytokines. Letra L, Santana I, Seiça R. Metab Brain Dis. 2014 Sep;29(3):563-8. doi: 10.1007/s11011-014-9501-z. Epub 2014 Feb 20. PMID: 24553879 DOI: 10.1007/s11011-014-9501-z

"Obesity has already been recognized as an important player in the pathogenesis of this type of dementia, independently of insulin resistance or other vascular risk factors."

"Although the exact underlying mechanisms are still unknown, adipocyte dysfunction and concomitant alteration in adipocyte-derived protein secretion seem to be involved, since these adipocytokines can cross the blood-brain barrier and influence cognitive-related structures."

"Interestingly, extensive research on the central effects of leptin in Alzheimer's disease-transgenic mice has demonstrated its capacity to enhance synaptic plasticity and strength, as well as to prevent beta-amyloid deposition and tau phosphorylation."

According to:
8. Alzheimer's disease risk, obesity and tau: is insulin resistance guilty? Blum D, Buée L. Expert Rev Neurother. 2013 May;13(5):461-3. doi: 10.1586/ern.13.35. PMID: 23621301 DOI: 10.1586/ern.13.35

"Obesity is thus undoubtedly a factor potentiating tau pathology but insulin resistance is probably not the missing link and factors involved remain to be identified."

"Contribution of dyslipidemia and cholesterol metabolism towards tau pathology during obesity is thus an interesting avenue to follow."

According to:
9. Obesity and dementia: adipokines interact with the brain. Arnoldussen IA1, Kiliaan AJ2, Gustafson DR3. Eur Neuropsychopharmacol. 2014 Dec;24(12):1982-99. Epub 2014 Mar 20. PMID: 24704273 PMCID: PMC4169761 DOI: 10.1016/j.euroneuro.2014.03.002

"Obesity has been associated with changes in brain structure, cognitive deficits, dementia and Alzheimer's disease."

"Adipokines, defined as hormones, cytokines and peptides secreted by adipose tissue, may have more widespread influence and functionality in the brain than previously thought. In this review, six adipokines, and their actions in the obese and non-obese conditions will be discussed."

- plasminogen activator inhibitor-1 (PAI-1),
- interleukin-6 (IL-6),
- tumor necrosis factors alpha (TNF-α),
- angiotensinogen (AGT),
- adiponectin
- leptin.

"Their functionality in the periphery, their ability to cross the blood brain barrier (BBB) and their influence on dementia processes within the brain will be discussed."

Polyphenols: ↓

The Short Story:
Defined: Polyphenols are a large group of phytochemicals which have evidence for their role in the prevention of degenerative diseases.

Summary: Great & wonderful!   Eat a ton of:
- Tea and coffee
- Flax and celery seed
- Pecans, almonds, walnut
- Berries, apples, peaches, orange
- Olives and olive oil.
- Mainly all the fruits, vegetables and nuts you can stand.

Lightning facts:
- "With **many** epidemiologic studies implying an association between **diet** and incidence of **dementia**, especially an association between a **greater plant source intake and lower incidence of cognitive impairment**, increasing scrutiny has focused on polyphenols as a possible disease-modifying factor [1]." [1.]
- Buckle up, polyphenols can: [2.]
    - **Alleviate** oxidation and free radicals.
    - **Increase** antioxidant and glutathione.
    - **Combat** inflammation.
    - **Inhibit** glutamate and excitotoxicity
    - **Help** fight the medications that **reduce** acetylcholine!

- o *Note: if the list above is confusing, there are chapters on each above, please feel free to read them for details.*
- "The pharmacological actions of curcumin, resveratrol and tea catechins have mainly been attributed to their antioxidant activity, interaction with cell signaling pathways, anti-inflammatory effect, chelation of metal ions, and neuroprotection." [4.]
- Current drugs help symptoms but don't stop the disease or heal it in any way. [5.]
- "In particular, the attention of researchers has been focused on phytochemical compounds that have shown antioxidative, anti-amyloidogenic, anti-inflammatory and anti-apoptotic properties and that could represent important resources in the discovery of drug candidates against dementia." [5.]

The Details:
According to:
1. A plant-tastic treatment for cognitive disorders. E.P. Cherniack Maturitas. 2012 Aug;72(4):265-6. doi: 10.1016/j.maturitas.2012.05.001. Epub 2012 May 31. The Geriatrics Institute, Division of Geriatrics and Gerontology, Geriatrics and Extended Care Services, and Geriatric Research, Education, and Clinical Center (GRECC) of the University of Miami Miller School of Medicine and the Miami VA Health Care System, Miami, FL 33125, United States Received: May 2, 2012; Published Online: May 23, 2012

"There has been a proliferation of recent interest in plant polyphenols as agents in the treatment of dementia."

" Many of these organic compounds, whose structure is characterized by multiple phenol rings, are found in a wide variety of fruits and vegetables [1]."

"With many epidemiologic studies implying an association between diet and incidence of dementia, especially an association between a greater plant source intake and lower incidence of cognitive impairment, increasing scrutiny has focused on polyphenols as a possible disease-modifying factor [1]."

According to:
2. Dietary Polyphenols as Potential Remedy for Dementia. Desai A. Adv Neurobiol. 2016;12:41-56. doi: 10.1007/978-3-319-28383-8_3. PMID: 27651247 DOI: 10.1007/978-3-319-28383-8_3

"Polyphenols, which constitute one such class of compounds, are dietary agents that are globally found in commonly consumed food."

"Many processes that are associated with the pathophysiology of dementia can be modulated by polyphenols."

"Polyphenolic compounds can alleviate oxidative stress by acting as direct scavengers of free radicals and clearing superoxide and hydroxyl radicals and by increasing the level of antioxidant enzymes such as glutathione peroxidase."

"Polyphenols can also combat inflammation by affecting transcription factors such as NF-κB."

"Some polyphenols may have the potential to inhibit excitotoxicity by regulating intracellular calcium ion concentration, inhibiting glutamate receptors and increasing glutamate reuptake at the synapse."

"The cognitive decline in dementia due to decreased availability of acetylcholine can also be countered by polyphenols that inhibit acetyl-cholinesterase activity."

According to:
3. Role of Plant Polyphenols in Alzheimer's Disease. Thenmozhi AJ, Manivasagam T, Essa MM. Adv Neurobiol. 2016;12:153-71. doi: 10.1007/978-3-319-28383-8_9. PMID: 27651253 DOI: 10.1007/978-3-319-28383-8_9

"Currently approved drugs for AD offer symptomatic relief without preventing the progression of the disease and having limited efficacy."

"Although several biological effects based on experimental studies could be scientifically explained, the way to bring natural polyphenols into routine clinical application against neurodegeneration seems to be long, because of its low average daily intake, poor availability and few adverse effects."

According to:
4. Polyphenols in dementia: From molecular basis to clinical trials. Molino S, Dossena M, Buonocore D, et al. Life Sci. 2016 Sep 15;161:69-77. Epub 2016 Aug 2. PMID: 27493077 DOI: 10.1016/j.lfs.2016.07.021

"In the last decade, polyphenols (particularly curcumin, resveratrol and tea catechins) have been under very close scrutiny as potential therapeutic agents for neurodegenerative diseases, diabetes, inflammatory diseases and aging."

"The pharmacological actions of curcumin, resveratrol and tea catechins have mainly been attributed to their antioxidant activity, interaction with cell signaling pathways, anti-inflammatory effect, chelation of metal ions, and neuroprotection."

According to:
5. Natural Phytochemicals in the Treatment and Prevention of Dementia: An Overview. Libro R, Giacoppo S, Soundara Rajan T, et al. Molecules. 2016 Apr 21;21(4):518. doi: 10.3390/molecules21040518. PMID: 27110749 DOI: 10.3390/molecules21040518

"There are different types of dementia, among which, Alzheimer's disease (AD), vascular dementia (VaD), dementia with Lewy bodies (DLB) and frontotemporal dementia (FTD) are the more common."

"In particular, the attention of researchers has been focused on phytochemical compounds that have shown antioxidative, anti-amyloidogenic, anti-inflammatory and anti-apoptotic properties and that could represent important resources in the discovery of drug candidates against dementia."

"In this review, we summarize the neuroprotective effects of the main phytochemicals belonging to the polyphenol, isothiocyanate, alkaloid and cannabinoid families in the prevention and treatment of the most common kinds of dementia."

Selenium: ↓

The Short Story:
Defined: Selenium is a chemical element, #34 on the periodic table of elements, considered a trace mineral for multiple human neurological functions.

Summary: When our selenium level becomes **depleted**, it begins a cascade of events which help promote dementia and Alzheimer's Disease.

Lightning facts:

- "**Optimal function** of these selenoenzymes requires **higher Se intake** than what is common in Europe and also higher intake than traditionally recommended." [1.]
- This study strengthens the hypothesis that selenium **helps to combat** oxidative stress which helps create Alzheimer's Disease. [2.]
- Selenium is important trace mineral in **regulating** brain function. [3.]
- Selenium aids and **strengthens** the brains **defense**. [3.]
- "A large body of studies suggests that selenium (Se), either as Se-containing compounds or as selenoproteins, may be beneficial in **reducing** Alzheimer's pathology." [4.]
- "Our findings suggest that the **deficiency** of Se may **contribute** to **cognitive decline** among aging people." [5.]

217

The Details:

According to:

1. Treatment strategies in Alzheimer's disease: a review with focus on selenium supplementation. Aaseth J, Alexander J, Bjørklund G, et al. Biometals. 2016 Oct;29(5):827-39. doi: 10.1007/s10534-016-9959-8. Epub 2016 Aug 16. PMID: 27530256 PMCID: PMC5034004 DOI: 10.1007/s10534-016-9959-8

"In recent years the main focus of AD research has been on the amyloid hypothesis, which postulates that extracellular precipitates of beta amyloid (Aβ) derived from amyloid precursor protein (APP) are responsible for the cognitive impairment seen in AD."

"Selenate is a potent inhibitor of tau hyperphosphorylation, a critical step in the formation of neurofibrillary tangles. Some selenium (Se) compounds e.g. selenoprotein P also appear to protect APP against excessive copper and iron deposition."

"Optimal function of these selenoenzymes requires higher Se intake than what is common in Europe and also higher intake than traditionally recommended."

"Supplementary treatment with N-acetylcysteine increases levels of the antioxidative cofactor glutathione and can mediate adjuvant protection."

According to:
2. Protective effect of selenium against aluminum chloride-induced Alzheimer's disease: behavioral and biochemical alterations in rats. Lakshmi BV1, Sudhakar M, Prakash KS. Biol Trace Elem Res. 2015 May;165(1):67-74. Epub 2015 Jan 23. PMID: 25613582 DOI: 10.1007/s12011-015-0229-3

"In present study, selenium was selected for evaluating effect of selenium on aluminum chloride (AlCl3)-induced Alzheimer's disease in rats."

"Therefore, this study strengthens the hypothesis that selenium helps to combat oxidative stress produced by accumulation of AlCl3 in the brain and helps in prophylaxis of Alzheimer's diseases."

According to:
3. Selenium in the Therapy of Neurological Diseases. Where is it Going? Dominiak A, Wilkaniec A, Wroczyński P, et al. Curr Neuropharmacol. 2016;14(3):282-99. PMID: 26549649 PMCID: PMC4857624

"Selenium (34Se), an antioxidant trace element, is an important regulator of brain function."

"Several selenoproteins are expressed in the brain, in which some of them, e.g. glutathione peroxidases (GPxs), thioredoxin reductases (TrxRs) or selenoprotein P (SelP), are strongly involved in antioxidant defence and in maintaining intercellular reducing conditions."

"Since increased oxidative stress has been implicated in neurological disorders, including Parkinson's disease, Alzheimer's disease, stroke, epilepsy and others, a growing body of evidence suggests that Se depletion followed by decreased activity of Se-dependent enzymes may be important factors connected with those pathologies."

According to:
4. Potential Roles of Selenium and Selenoproteins in the Prevention of Alzheimer's Disease. Du X, Wang C, Liu Q. Curr Top Med Chem. 2016;16(8):835-48. PMID: 26311427

"A large body of studies suggests that selenium (Se), either as Se-containing compounds or as selenoproteins, may be beneficial in reducing Alzheimer's pathology."

"Se is involved in most of the molecular pathways that are important in the progression of AD."

According to:
5. Selenium status in elderly: relation to cognitive decline. Rita Cardoso B1, Silva Bandeira V2, Jacob-Filho W3, Franciscato Cozzolino SM2. J Trace Elem Med Biol. 2014 Oct;28(4):422-6. Epub 2014 Aug 28. PMID: 25220532 DOI: 10.1016/j.jtemb.2014.08.009

"Thus we aimed to measure selenium (Se) status in Alzheimer's disease (AD) and mild cognitive impairment (MCI) elderly and compared them with a control group (CG)."

"It is observed that erythrocyte Se decreases as cognition function does."

"Our findings suggest that the deficiency of Se may contribute to cognitive decline among aging people."

According to:
6. Selenium treatment significantly inhibits tumor necrosis factor-α-induced cell death and tau hyperphosphorylation in neuroblastoma cells. Lee YJ, Kim JE, Kwak MH, et al. Mol Med Rep. 2014 Oct;10(4):1869-74. Epub 2014 Aug 4. PMID: 25109896 DOI: 10.3892/mmr.2014.2442

"The hyperphosphorylation of the protein tau disrupts its normal function on regulating axonal transport and leads to the accumulation of neurofibrillary tangles (NFT), which are involved in the pathogenesis of Alzheimer's disease (AD)."

"Overall, these results provide strong evidence that sodium selenite (selenium) can inhibit cell death and tau phosphorylation induced by TNF-α in neuroblastoma cells, through the inhibition GSK-3β and Akt phosphorylation."

Statin: ↕

The Short Story:
Defined: Statins are a group of drugs that act to reduce levels of fats, including triglycerides and cholesterol, in the blood by altering the enzyme activity in the liver that produces lipids.

Summary: From some reports suggesting statins are neutral or beneficial to studies that have no difference or another study suggesting it makes no overall difference. Still more calling statins no significances! Plus, there are risks of cognitive impairment and cerebral vascular disease.

Lightning facts:

- "Despite several reports of **statin-associated cognitive impairment,** this adverse effect remains a rare occurrence among the totality of the literature." [1.]

- "Conversely, in the **majority** of randomized controlled trials and observational studies, statins were found to have either a **neutral** or **beneficial** effect on cognition." [1.]

- "This study found **no difference** in the risk of dementia among current and former users of statins as compared with nonusers in an already at-risk HF population." [3.]

- "There was **no overall** effect of statin exposure on cerebral structural indices." [5.]

- "There were **no significant differences** between the statins and placebo groups regarding the main outcomes, secondary outcomes, or adverse events."
  6.

- "**Most** of the studies **ignored** or **downplayed risk** factors for **cerebral vascular disease.**" 6.

The Details:
According to:

1. Is statin-associated cognitive impairment clinically relevant? A narrative review and clinical recommendations. Rojas-Fernandez CH, Cameron JC. Ann Pharmacother. 2012 Apr;46(4):549-57 Epub 2012 Apr 3. PMID: 22474137 [PubMed - indexed for MEDLINE]

"To explore the impact of statin use on cognition."

"A literature search was performed using MEDLINE (1950-November 2011), EMBASE (1980-November 2011), and the Cochrane Library (1960-November 2011)."

"One randomized controlled trial demonstrated that simvastatin impaired some measures of cognition compared to placebo. Conversely, in the majority of randomized controlled trials and observational studies, statins were found to have either a neutral or beneficial effect on cognition."

"Despite several reports of statin-associated cognitive impairment, this adverse effect remains a rare occurrence among the totality of the literature."

According to:
2. Effects of vascular risk factors, statins, and antihypertensive drugs on PiB deposition in cognitively normal subjects. Glodzik L, Rusinek H, Kamer A, et al. Alzheimers Dement (Amst). 2016 Apr 19;2:95-104. eCollection 2016. PMID: 27239540 PMCID: PMC4879519 DOI: 10.1016/j.dadm.2016.02.007

"Hypertension, hypercholesterolemia, and obesity increase the risk of dementia."

"Prospective studies should confirm effects of drugs and increased body weight on amyloid accumulation and establish whether they translate into measurable clinical outcomes. Women may be more susceptible to harmful effects of obesity."

According to:
3. Use of Statins and Risk of Dementia in Heart Failure: A Retrospective Cohort Study. Chitnis AS, Aparasu RR, Chen H, et al. Drugs Aging. 2015 Sep;32(9):743-54. PMID: 26363909 DOI: 10.1007/s40266-015-0295-4

"Heart failure (HF) is associated with an increased risk of dementia, and studies show that dyslipidemia may be involved in the pathogenesis of dementia."

"The present study examines the effectiveness of statins to prevent dementia in HF patients."

"The study included a total of 8062 HF patients (mean age 74.47 ± 9.21 years), of whom 1135 (14.08%) were diagnosed with dementia during a median follow-up of 22 months."

"This study found no difference in the risk of dementia among current and former users of statins as compared with nonusers in an already at-risk HF population."

According to:
4. Do statins prevent Alzheimer's disease? A narrative review. Daneschvar HL, Aronson MD, Smetana GW. Eur J Intern Med. 2015 Nov;26(9):666-9. Epub 2015 Sep 2. PMID: 26342722 DOI: 10.1016/j.ejim.2015.08.012

"Cholesterol related pathways might play a role in the pathogenesis of Alzheimer's disease. Treatment with 3-hydroxy-3-methylglutaryl-coenzyme A (HMG-CoA) reductase inhibitors (statins) has been suggested to promote the prevention of Alzheimer's disease."

According to
5. Statins and brain integrity in older adults: secondary analysis of the Health ABC study. Nadkarni NK, Perera S, Hanlon JT, Alzheimers Dement. 2015 Oct;11(10):1202-11. Epub 2015 Jan 12. PMID: 25592659 PMCID: PMC4499493 DOI: 10.1016/j.jalz.2014.11.003

"We examined whether statins are associated with better cerebral white (WM) and gray matter (GM) indices in community-dwelling elders."

"There was no overall effect of statin exposure on cerebral structural indices."

"Statins may benefit WM in older adults vulnerable to dementia."

According to
6. Statins for Treating Alzheimer's Disease: Truly Ineffective? Liang T1, Li R, Cheng O. Eur Neurol. 2015;73(5-6):360-6. Epub 2015 May 28. PMID: 26021802 DOI: 10.1159/000382128

"To evaluate the efficacy and safety of statins in the treatment of AD."

"Four studies (1,127 participants) involving patients with a diagnosis of probable or possible AD were included. There were no significant differences between the statins and placebo groups regarding the main outcomes, secondary outcomes, or adverse events."

"Most of the studies ignored or downplayed risk factors for cerebral vascular disease."

Stroke: ↑

The Short Story:
Defined: A stroke is when the blood supply to part of your brain is interrupted or severely reduced.

Summary: The risk of dementia from a stroke is from 6 to upwards of 30 percent based on where you live and what type of stoke you have.

> *Authors note:* Do everything you can to prevent a stroke from happening to eating better, losing weight and exercising.

Lightning facts:
- Following a stroke, your chance of having **higher** rate of **dementia** and **post-stroke cognitive impairment** is between **46-61%**. [Scandanavia] [1.]
  - *Author's note:* this is where you read the previous chapters and get to work making changes to lower things that bring you further risk and increase the things to bring this high risk down.
- "Current evidence suggests that **25-30% of ischemic stroke survivors** develop immediate or delayed vascular cognitive impairment or vascular dementia." [Japan] [2.]
- "Cognitive impairment is a common sequel to stroke; the rate of **post-stroke dementia is 6% to 30%**." [Hong Kong] [3.]

- **Ischaemic stroke** victims have **25-30%** develop immediate or delayed vascular congnitive impairment or dementia. [5.]

The Details:
According to:
1. Cognitive function in stroke survivors: A 10-year follow-up study. Delavaran H, Jönsson AC, Lövkvist H, et al. Acta Neurol Scand. 2016 Nov 1. PMID: 27804110 DOI: 10.1111/ane.12709

"Post-stroke cognitive impairment (PSCI) has considerable impact on patients and society."

"Of 145 stroke survivors after 10 years, 127 participated. Mini-Mental State Examination (MMSE) showed PSCI in 46%, whereas Montreal Cognitive Assessment (MoCA) displayed PSCI in 61%."

Post-stroke cognitive impairment was prevalent among 10-year stroke survivors, and the odds of having severe cognitive impairment were higher among the stroke survivors compared to non-stroke persons.

According to:
2. [Post Stroke Dementia]. [Article in Japanese] Ihara M. Brain Nerve. 2016 Jul;68(7):743-51. PMID: 27395459 DOI: 10.11477/mf.1416200506

"Post-stroke dementia (PSD) is a clinical entity that encompasses all types of dementia following an index stroke."

"Current evidence suggests that 25-30% of ischemic stroke survivors develop immediate or delayed vascular cognitive impairment or vascular dementia."

"Published clinical trials have not been promising and there is little information on whether PSD can be prevented using pharmacological agents."

"Control of vascular disease risk and prevention of recurrent strokes are key to reducing the burden of cognitive decline and post-stroke dementia."

According to:
3. Detection of amyloid plaques in patients with post-stroke dementia. Mok VC, Liu WY, Wong A. Hong Kong Med J. 2016 Feb;22 Suppl 2:S40-2. PMID: 26908343

"Cognitive impairment is a common sequel to stroke; the rate of post-stroke dementia is 6% to 30%."

"Alzheimer's disease treatment (eg acetylcholinesterase inhibitors) may be more beneficial in patients with mixed dementia than in those with pure vascular dementia."

"Concurrent amyloid pathology is found in about one fifth of patients with stroke or transient ischaemic attack and dementia; it can exert a negative longterm impact upon cognitive progression."

According to:
4. Urine Formaldehyde Predicts Cognitive Impairment in Post-Stroke Dementia and Alzheimer's Disease. Tong Z, Wang W, Luo W, et al. J Alzheimers Dis. 2016 Oct 14. PMID: 27802225 DOI: 10.3233/JAD-160357

"Here, we investigated the relationship between morning urine formaldehyde concentration and cognitive impairment in patients with post-stroke dementia (PSD) or AD in this cross-sectional survey for 7 years."

"The findings suggest that measuring the concentration of formaldehyde in overnight fasting urine could be used as a potentially noninvasive method for evaluating the likelihood of ensuing cognitive impairment or dementia."

According to:
5. Stroke injury, cognitive impairment and vascular dementia. Kalaria RN, Akinyemi R, Ihara M. Biochim Biophys Acta. 2016 May;1862(5):915-25. Epub 2016 Jan 22. PMID: 26806700 PMCID: PMC4827373 DOI: 10.1016/j.bbadis.2016.01.015

"The global burden of ischaemic strokes is almost 4-fold greater than haemorrhagic strokes. Current evidence suggests that 25-30% of ischaemic stroke survivors develop immediate or delayed vascular cognitive impairment (VCI) or vascular dementia (VaD)."

Turmeric: ↓

The Short Story:
Defined: The ginger family has a rhizome plant called Curcuma domestica.

Summary: Turmeric has been used over 2000 years in Asia and just recently it has a lot press in the US. Patients have asked and taking this mixed with black pepper increases and boosts its anti-inflammatory effects. Take up to one teaspoon a day.

Lightning facts:
- Turmeric / curcumin have the bulk of the research in polyphenol research and is **proven** helper to **fight** Alzheimer's Disease and dementia amongst other diseases. [1]
- Turmeric along with vitamin E & saffron **prevent** an **enzyme** from **destroying** Acetylcholine (see the medicine chapter) which can help decrease dementia and Alzheimer's. [2]
- **Turmeric works better than curcumin alone!** [3]
- Polyphenol that provide substantial neuroprotective benefits. [4]
  - Herbs: "**Green tea, turmeric**, Salvia miltiorrhiza, and Panax **ginseng**,"
  - Spices: "**Cinnamon, ginger, rosemary, sage**, salvia herbs, Chinese celery and many others."
- Curcumin **binds** in a way to the plaques relate to the patient in a **non-toxic aggregate**. [5]

- "Co-ingestion of **turmeric** with **white bread** increases working memory independent of body fatness, glycaemia, insulin, or AD biomarkers." [6.]
- **Curcumin has dangers at high doses.** [7.]

The Details:
According to:
1. Plant-derived health: the effects of turmeric and curcuminoids. Bengmark S, Mesa MD, Gil A. Nutr Hosp. 2009 May-Jun;24(3):273-81. PMID: 19721899 [PubMed - indexed for MEDLINE]

"Examples of such polyphenols are isothiocyanates in cabbage and broccoli, epigallocatechin in green tee, capsaicin in chili peppers, chalones, rutin and naringenin in apples, resveratrol in red wine and fresh peanuts and curcumin/curcuminoids in turmeric."

"Most diseases are maintained by a sustained discreet but obvious increased systemic inflammation."

"To the polyphenols with a bulk of experimental documentation belong the curcuminoid family and especially its main ingredient, curcumin."

"It is suggested that supply of polyphenols and particularly curcuminoids might be value as complement to pharmaceutical treatment, but also prebiotic treatment, in conditions proven to be rather therapy-resistant such as Crohn's, long-stayed patients in intensive care units, but also in conditions such as cancer, liver cirrhosis, chronic renal disease, chronic obstructive lung disease, diabetes and Alzheimer's disease."

According to:
2. Vitamin E, Turmeric and Saffron in Treatment of Alzheimer's Disease. Adalier N, Parker H. Antioxidants (Basel). 2016 Oct 25;5(4). pii: E40. PMID: 27792130 DOI: 10.3390/antiox5040040

"The paper highlights use of vitamin E, turmeric and saffron for an alternative antioxidant therapy approach."

"Clinical studies report their therapeutic abilities as protective agents for nerve cells against free radical damage, moderating acetylcholinesterase (AChE) activity and reducing neurodegeneration, which are found as key factors in Alzheimer's."

According to:
3. Therapeutic potential of turmeric in Alzheimer's disease: curcumin or curcuminoids? Ahmed T, Gilani AH. Phytother Res. 2014 Apr;28(4):517-25. Epub 2013 Jul 19. PMID: 23873854 DOI: 10.1002/ptr.5030

"Turmeric possesses multiple medicinal uses including treatment for AD. Curcuminoids, a mixture of curcumin, demethoxycurcumin, and bisdemethoxycurcumin, are vital constituents of turmeric."

"Therefore, it is emphasized in this review that each component of the curcuminoid mixture plays a distinct role in making curcuminoid mixture useful in AD, and hence, the curcuminoid mixture represents turmeric in its medicinal value better than curcumin alone."

According to:
4. Brain Food for Alzheimer-Free Ageing: Focus on Herbal Medicines. Hügel HM. Adv Exp Med Biol. 2015;863:95-116. PMID: 26092628 DOI: 10.1007/978-3-319-18365-7_5

"Therefore, lifestyle choices are paramount to leading either a brain-derived or a brain-deprived life."

"Plants can be considered as chemical factories that manufacture huge numbers of diverse bioactive substances, many of which have the potential to provide substantial neuroprotective benefits."

"Medicinal herbs and health food supplements have been widely used in Asia since over 2,000 years."

"Many herbs with anti-amyloidogenic activity, including those containing polyphenolic constituents such as green tea, turmeric, Salvia miltiorrhiza, and Panax ginseng, are presented."

"Also covered in this review are extracts from kitchen spices including cinnamon, ginger, rosemary, sage, salvia herbs, Chinese celery and many others some of which are commonly used in herbal combinations and represent highly promising therapeutic natural compounds against AD."

According to:
5. Curcumin Binding to Beta Amyloid: A Computational Study. Rao PP, Mohamed T, Teckwani K, et al. PMID: 25776887 DOI: 10.1111/cbdd.12552

"Curcumin, a chemical constituent present in the spice turmeric, is known to prevent the aggregation of amyloid peptide implicated in the pathophysiology of Alzheimer's disease."

"Analysis of MD trajectories of curcumin bound to full-length Aβ fibril shows good stability with minimum Cα-atom RMSD shifts."

"These results show that curcumin binding to Aβ shifts the equilibrium in the aggregation pathway by promoting the formation of non-toxic aggregates."

According to:
6. Turmeric improves post-prandial working memory in pre-diabetes independent of insulin. Lee MS, Wahlqvist ML, Chou YC, et al. Asia Pac J Clin Nutr. 2014;23(4):581-91. PMID: 25516316

"Cognitive impairment develops with pre-diabetes and dementia is a complication of diabetes."

"Natural products like turmeric and cinnamon may ameliorate the underlying pathogenesis."

"No interaction between turmeric and cinnamon was detected."

"WM increased from 2.6 to 2.9 out of 3.0 (p=0.05) with turmeric, but was unchanged with cinnamon. WM improvement was inversely associated with insulin resistance (r=-0.418, p<0.01), but not with AD biomarkers."

"Co-ingestion of turmeric with white bread increases working memory independent of body fatness, glycaemia, insulin, or AD biomarkers."

According to:
7. Neuroprotective properties of curcumin in Alzheimer's disease--merits and limitations. Chin D, Huebbe P, Pallauf K, et al. Curr Med Chem. 2013;20(32):3955-85. PMID: 23931272

"One popular candidate is curcumin or diferuloylmethane, a polyphenolic compound that is the main curcuminoid found in Curcuma longa (family Zingiberaceae)."

"In recent years, curcumin has been reported to possess anti-amyloidogenic, antiinflammatory, anti-oxidative, and metal chelating properties that may result in potential neuroprotective effects."

"Furthermore, although many have reported that curcumin possesses a relatively low toxicity profile, curcumin applied at high doses, which is not uncommon practice in many in vivo and clinical studies, may present certain dangers that in our opinion have not been addressed sufficiently."

Vitamin B12: ↓

The Short Story:
Defined: Cobalamin, is one of the eight B vitamins responsible for proper functioning in of the nervous system, brain tissue, memory, and proper red cell development to name a few.

Summary: **Keep your B12 high**!!! Once it get's low with a higher homocysteine your risks start to sky rocket! While adding it to dementia or cognitive function decline will not help, keeping it high when we are healthy will certainly shift your risk lower!

Lightning facts:
- "Vitamin B12 is **essential** for **DNA synthesis** and for **cellular energy** production." [1]
- A meta-analysis and review identified a correlation between tHcy and Alzheimer's Disease, and suggested the effect was **due to lower levels of vitamins B12, B6 and folate** [76]." [1]
- "A nutritional-based strategy has been proposed in order to **improve** cognitive performance of Alzheimer's disease (AD) patients. The strategy requires **daily** dietary supplementation with **magnesium** (Mg), **folic acid**, and vitamins **B6** and **B12**, daily consumption of **silicic acid-rich mineral** water in order to **lower** the body burden of Al, and several plasma exchange procedures in order to replace Aβ-bound albumin with fresh albumin." [2]

- Ok, so when homocysteine, Vit B 12 and folate are all normal we have a risk of dementia / Alzheimer's Disease of 1.0. When our blood work shows **high** homocysteine, **low** B-12 and **any** folate value we have **30 times the risk!!** [3.] *See chart on p. 241*
- "Second, data suggests that **high** Hcy and **low** folate levels may correlate with **increased** risk of AD occurrence." [4.]
- "Similarly, folic acid alone or vitamins B in combination are unable to stabilize or slow decline in cognition, function, behavior, and global change of AD patients." [5.]

The Details:
According to:
1. Vitamin B12 in Health and Disease Fiona O'Leary and Samir Samman* Nutrients. 2010 Mar; 2(3): 299–316. Published online 2010 Mar 5. doi: 10.3390/nu2030299 PMCID: PMC3257642

"Vitamin B12 is essential for DNA synthesis and for cellular energy production."

"Vitamin B12 deficiency is common, mainly due to limited dietary intake of animal foods or malabsorption of the vitamin. Vegetarians are at risk of vitamin B12 deficiency as are other groups with low intakes of animal foods or those with restrictive dietary patterns."

"A deficiency of vitamin B12 and the interruption of this reaction leads to the development of megaloblastic anaemia."

"Gastritis or inflammation of the gastric mucosa increases with age and results in a reduction, or in some cases, complete loss of the acid required to cleave vitamin B12 from protein."

"The monitoring of vitamin B12 concentrations is recommended for patients undergoing prolonged PPI treatment, in recognition that the bioavailability of food-bound vitamin B12 may be compromised [3]."

"Metformin is a biguanide used for the treatment of non-insulin dependent diabetes and some patients taking this medication develop megaloblastic anaemia [34,35]."

"In older people with low vitamin B12 status, a high serum folate concentration was associated with increased odds of cognitive impairment, but in subjects with normal vitamin B12 status, high serum folate was found to be protective against cognitive impairment [74]."

"A meta-analysis and review identified a correlation between tHcy and Alzheimer's Disease, and suggested the effect was due to lower levels of vitamins B12, B6 and folate [76]."

According to:
2. A multipronged, nutritional-based strategy for managing Alzheimer's disease. Glick JL, McMillan PA. Med Hypotheses. 2016 Jun;91:98-102. doi: 10.1016/j.mehy.2016.04.007. Epub 2016 Apr 8. PMID: 27142155 DOI: 10.1016/j.mehy.2016.04.007

"A nutritional-based strategy has been proposed in order to improve cognitive performance of Alzheimer's disease (AD) patients. The strategy requires daily dietary supplementation with magnesium (Mg), folic acid, and vitamins B6 and B12, daily consumption of silicic acid-rich mineral water in order to lower the body burden of Al, and several plasma exchange procedures in order to replace Aβ-bound albumin with fresh albumin."

"However, for the following reasons the combination of all four therapeutic approaches may have a synergistic effect on improving cognitive performance of AD patients."

According to:
3. Associations between Alzheimer's disease and blood homocysteine, vitamin B12, and folate: a case-control study. Chen H, Liu S, Ji L, et al. Curr Alzheimer Res. 2015;12(1):88-94. PMID: 25523421

"There is a growing focus on nutritional therapy for Alzheimer's disease (AD), and controversy exists regarding the association between AD and homocysteine (Hcy), vitamin B12, and folate levels."

Homocy	Vit B12	Folate	*Increased Odds of AD*
Normal	Normal	Normal	1.0
Normal	Low	Normal	4.6
Normal	Low	Low	4.3
High	Normal	Low	17.0
High	**Low**	**Any**	**30.5**

"Vitamin B12 was directly associated with AD. The combination of high Hcy, low vitamin B12, and any folate level represented the poorest association with AD."

According to:
4. Associations between Homocysteine, Folic Acid, Vitamin B12 and Alzheimer's Disease: Insights from Meta-Analyses. Shen L, Ji HF. J Alzheimers Dis. 2015;46(3):777-90. PMID: 25854931 DOI: 10.3233/JAD-150140

"The associations between homocysteine (Hcy), folic acid, and vitamin B12 and Alzheimer's disease (AD) have gained much interest, while remaining controversial."

"First, AD patients may have higher level of Hcy, and lower levels of folate and vitamin B12 in plasma than controls."

"Second, data suggests that high Hcy and low folate levels may correlate with increased risk of AD occurrence."

"The comprehensive meta-analyses not only confirmed higher Hcy, lower folic acid, and vitamin B12 levels in AD patients than controls, but also implicated that high Hcy and low folic acid levels may be risk factors of AD."

According to:
5. Efficacy of vitamins B supplementation on mild cognitive impairment and Alzheimer's disease: a systematic review and meta-analysis. Li MM, Yu JT, Wang HF, et al. Curr Alzheimer Res. 2014;11(9):844-52. PMID: 25274113

"The aim of this study was to systematically review and quantitatively synthesize the efficacy of treatment with vitamins B supplementation in slowing the rate of cognitive, behavioral, functional and global decline in individuals with MCI or AD."

"Similarly, folic acid alone or vitamins B in combination are unable to stabilize or slow decline in cognition, function, behavior, and global change of AD patients."

Vitamin D: ↓

The Short Story:
Defined: A group of fat-soluable secosteroids, found in liver and fish oils, essential for responsible for increasing intestinal absorption of calcium, iron, magnesium, phosphate, and zinc.

Summary: Easy, economical, affordable. Check your blood lab or get the test and then **take** at least 5,000 units of Vitamin D3.

Lightning facts:
- **Decreased** vitamin D are associated with dementia and Alzheimer's Disease. [1.]
- "**Hypo**vitaminosis D, a common condition in older adults, is associated with brain changes and dementia." [2.]
- "Some of the <u>neurosteroid</u> <u>actions</u> of vitamin D include **regulation of calcium** homeostasis, **clearance** of amyloid-β peptide, **antioxidant** and **anti-inflammatory** effects, and possible **protection** against the neurodegenerative mechanisms associated with Alzheimer's disease (AD)." [3.]
- "In conclusion, vitamin D **supplementation** caused **significant** improvement in the cognitive performance in subjects with senile dementia." [4.]
- "**Vitamin D stimulates macrophages [the primary cell of the innate immune response], which increases the clearance of amyloid plaques, a hallmark of AD**" [6.]

- Vitamin D blood levels and risks. [6.]

Sufficient > 50 nmol/L	Deficient 25 – 50 nmol/L	Severely deficient < 25 nmol/L
	+ 53% dementia	**+ 125% dementia**
	+ 69% Alzheimer's	**+ 122% Alzheimer's**

The Details:
According to:
1. Genetically decreased vitamin D and risk of Alzheimer disease. Mokry LE, Ross S, Morris JA, et al. Neurology. 2016 Nov 16. PMID: 27856775 DOI: 10.1212/WNL.0000000000003430.

"To test whether genetically decreased vitamin D levels are associated with Alzheimer disease (AD) using mendelian randomization (MR), a method that minimizes bias due to confounding or reverse causation."

"We measured the effect of each of these single nucleotide polymorphisms (SNPs) on 25OHD levels in the Canadian Multicentre Osteoporosis Study (CaMos; N = 2,347) and obtained the corresponding effect estimates for each SNP on AD risk from the International Genomics of Alzheimer's Project (N = 17,008 AD cases and 37,154 controls)."

"MR analyses demonstrated that a 1-SD decrease in natural log-transformed 25OHD increased AD risk by 25% (odds ratio 1.25, 95% confidence interval 1.03-1.51, p = 0.021)."

"Our results provide evidence supporting 25OHD as a causal risk factor for AD."

According to:
2. Vitamin D and cognition in older adults: international consensus guidelines. Annweiler C, Dursun E, Féron F, et al. Geriatr Psychol Neuropsychiatr Vieil. 2016 Sep 1;14(3):265-73. PMID: 27651008 DOI: 10.1684/pnv.2016.0613

"Hypovitaminosis D, a common condition in older adults, is associated with brain changes and dementia."

"International experts met at the invitational summit on "Vitamin D and cognition in older adults" in Boston, MA, July 2013. Based upon literature and expert opinion, the task force focused on key questions on the role of vitamin D in Alzheimer disease and related disorders."

"Experts reached agreement that hypovitaminosis D increases the risk of cognitive decline and dementia in older adults, may alter the clinical presentation as a consequence of related comorbidities, but should not be used thus far as a diagnostic or prognostic biomarker of Alzheimer disease due to lack of specificity and insufficient evidence."

According to:
3. Vitamin D in dementia prevention. Annweiler C1,2,3. Ann N Y Acad Sci. 2016 Mar;1367(1):57-63. PMID: 27116242 DOI: 10.1111/nyas.13058

"Beyond effects on bone health, vitamin D exerts effects on a variety of target organs, including the brain."

"Some of the neurosteroid actions of vitamin D include regulation of calcium homeostasis, clearance of amyloid-β peptide, antioxidant and anti-inflammatory effects, and possible protection against the neurodegenerative mechanisms associated with Alzheimer's disease (AD)."

"... several nonrandomized controlled studies have found that older adults experienced cognitive improvements after 1-15 months of vitamin D supplementation. Therefore, it appears crucial to maintain vitamin D concentrations at sufficiently high levels in order to slow, prevent, or improve neurocognitive decline."

According to:
4. Role of Vitamin-D in the prevention and treatment of Alzheimer's disease. Gangwar AK, Rawat A, Tiwari S, et al. Indian J Physiol Pharmacol. 2015 Jan-Mar;59(1):94-9. PMID: 26571990

"Alzheimer's disease is the most common form of age related cognitive impairment."

"Aim of the present study was to see the effect of vitamin D on cognitive function in elderly."

"In conclusion, vitamin D supplementation caused significant improvement in the cognitive performance in subjects with senile dementia."

According to:
5. Vitamin D and Alzheimer's Disease: Neurocognition to Therapeutics. Banerjee A, Khemka VK, Ganguly A, et al. Int J Alzheimers Dis. 2015;2015:192747. Epub 2015 Aug 17. PMID: 26351614 PMCID: PMC4553343 DOI: 10.1155/2015/192747

"The sporadic form of AD accounts for nearly 90% of the patients developing this disease."

"Accumulating evidences suggested a significant association between vitamin D deficiency, dementia, and AD."

"This review encompasses the beneficial role of vitamin D in neurocognition and optimal brain health along with epidemiological evidence of the high prevalence of hypovitaminosis D among aged and AD population."

According to:
6. Vitamin D and the risk of dementia and Alzheimer disease. Neurology August 6, 2014 [epub] Thomas J. Littlejohns, William E. Henley, Iain A. Lang, et al. From the University of Exeter Medical School, Exeter, UK

"This is the first large, prospective, population-based study assessment of dementia and Alzheimer's disease (AD) and the relationship with vitamin D concentrations."

"They assessed 1,658 elderly ambulatory adults by measuring serum 25-hydroxyvitamin D (25 (OH) D) concentrations. Subjects were followed for a mean of 5.6 years. This constitutes 9,317.5 person-years of followup;

171 participants developed all-cause dementia, including 102 cases of Alzheimer disease."

- Sufficient vitamin D concentration was > 50 nmol/L [>20 ng/ml]
- Deficient vitamin D concentration was between 25 - 50 nmol/L [10-20 ng/ml]
  o The increased risk for all-cause dementia in those who were deficient 25(OH)D was 53%.
  o The increased risk for Alzheimer's disease in those who were deficient 25(OH)D was 69%.
- Severely deficient vitamin D concentration was < 25 nmol/L [< 10 ng/ml]
  o The increased risk for all-cause dementia in those who were severely deficient 25(OH)D was 125%.
  o The increased risk for Alzheimer's disease in those who were severely deficient 25(OH)D was 122%.

"Vitamin D increases the phagocytic clearance of amyloid plaques by stimulating macrophages and reduces amyloid-induced cytotoxicity and apoptosis in primary cortical neurons."

Vitamin D stimulates macrophages [the primary cell of the innate immune response], which increases the clearance of amyloid plaques, a hallmark of AD.

This study and many others we have reviewed support that most people should be supplementing with a least 5,000 IU of vitamin D3 / day.

Walking: ↓

The Short Story:
Defined: To go for a walk, greater than 20 minutes.

Summary: Walking **helps** executive function, functional capacity and can slow cognitive decline even in a person with dementia

Lightning facts:
- "**Daily** steps, executive function, subjective memory complaints, functional capacity and 5-m maximum walking time **significantly improved** during the intervention period" [1]
- "This study shows that a physical activity program can **slow** cognitive decline and **improve** quality of walking in elderly persons suffering from dementia." [2]

The Details:
According to:
1. Prevention of cognitive and physical decline by enjoyable walking-habituation program based on brain-activating rehabilitation. Murai T, Yamaguchi T, Maki Y, et al. Geriatr Gerontol Int. 2016 Jun;16(6):701-8. Epub 2015 Jun 16. PMID: 26082004 DOI: 10.1111/ggi.12541

"We carried out a 12-week intervention, consisting of an enjoyable walking-habituation program based on five principles of brain-activating rehabilitation: pleasant atmosphere, interactive communication, social roles, praising each other and errorless support."

"The program, once a week for 90 min, was carried out in small groups."

"Daily steps, executive function, subjective memory complaints, functional capacity and 5-m maximum walking time significantly improved during the intervention period (after observation to after intervention) compared with the observation period (before the observation period to after observation)."

According to:
2. Effects of a physical training programme on cognitive function and walking efficiency in elderly persons with dementia. Kemoun G, Thibaud M, Roumagne N, et al. Geriatr Cogn Disord. 2010;29(2):109-14. Epub 2010 Feb 11. PMID: 20150731 DOI: 10.1159/000272435

"To study the effects of physical stimulation based on walking exercises, equilibrium and endurance on cognitive function and walking efficiency in patients with dementia."

"Randomized controlled trial including 31 subjects suffering from dementia (age: 81.8 +/- 5.3 years)."

"After the 15 weeks of rehabilitation, the subjects from the intervention group improved their overall ERFC score (p < 0.01), while those in the control group decreased their overall ERFC score."

"This study shows that a physical activity programme can slow cognitive decline and improve quality of walking in elderly persons suffering from dementia."

Zinc: ↓

The Short Story:
Defined: Atomic number 30, it is key for neuroprotection and key brain functions.

Summary: A number of studies suggest a therapeutic dose of **supplemental** zinc is 15-25 mg/day but taking too much zinc may produce a deficiency of copper.

Lightning facts:
- Just eating garlic or onions to grains can increase the bioavailability of zinc when combined by 50% or more. [1.]
- "Unexpected significantly **low serum zinc** concentrations were found in patients with Alzheimer's disease and Parkinson's disease compared to age matched controls." [2.]
- "**Zinc** is a key component to numerous **neuroprotective** enzymes, including those responsible for degradation of Alzheimer's amyloid B." [3.]
- "Furthermore, **Zn plays a central role** in ischemia-induced neuronal death and the pathogenesis of vascular dementia." [4.]
- "Our meta-analysis results showed that **serum zinc was significantly lower in AD patients.** Our replication and meta-analysis results showed that **serum copper was significantly higher in AD** patients than in healthy controls." [5.]

The Details:
According to:
1. Higher bioaccessibility of iron and zinc from food grains in the presence of garlic and onion. Gautam S, Platel K, Srinivasan K. J Agric Food Chem. 2010 Jul 28;58(14):8426-9. doi: 10.1021/jf100716t. PMID: 20597543

"Bioavailability of micronutrients iron and zinc is particularly low from plant foods."

"In this context, we examined the influence of exogenously added garlic and onion on the bioaccessibility of iron and zinc from food grains."

"The two spices similarly enhanced the bioaccessibility of zinc from the food grains, the extent of increase in cereals ranging from 10.4% to 159.4% and in pulses from 9.8% to 49.8%."

According to:
2. Mutation Research/Fundamental and Molecular Mechanisms of Mutagenesis. Bruce N. Ames, University of California, Berkeley Volume 475, Issues 1-2, 18 April 2001, Pages 7-20

"Results showed significantly lower blood zinc in patients with Alzheimer's and patients with Parkinson's than in controls."

"Unexpected significantly low serum zinc concentrations were found in patients with Alzheimer's disease and Parkinson's disease compared to age matched controls."

"Zinc in the hippocampus plays an important role as a synaptic neurotransmitter that modulates N-methyl-D-aspartic acid (NMDA) receptor activity that limits neuroexcitation." Eg. Zinc protects nerves from damange.

According to:
3. Subclinical Zinc Deficiency in Alzheimer's Disease and Parkinson's Disease. American Journal of Alzheimer's Disease and Other Dementias. George J. Brewer, Steve H. Kanzer, Earl A. Zimmerman, et al. September 14, 2010; Vol. 25; No. 7; pp. 572-575

"Zinc is a key component to numerous neuroprotective enzymes, including those responsible for degradation of Alzheimer's amyloid B."

"Patients with Alzheimer's have a significantly lower level of zinc in their cerebral spinal fluid."

According to:
4. Disruption of zinc homeostasis and the pathogenesis of senile dementia. Kawahara M, Mizuno D, Koyama H, et al. Metallomics. 2014 Feb;6(2):209-19. PMID: 24247360 DOI: 10.1039/c3mt00257h

"Zinc (Zn) is an essential trace element that is abundantly present in the brain. Although Zn plays crucial roles in learning and memory, numerous studies have indicated that the disruption of Zn homeostasis, namely both depletion and excess Zn, causes severe damage to neurons and is linked with various neurodegenerative diseases including Alzheimer's disease and vascular dementia."

"Furthermore, Zn plays a central role in ischemia-induced neuronal death and the pathogenesis of vascular dementia."

According to:
5. Protective substances against zinc-induced neuronal death after ischemia: carnosine as a target for drug of vascular type of dementia. Kawahara M, Konoha K, Nagata T, et al. Recent Pat CNS Drug Discov. 2007 Jun;2(2):145-9. PMID: 18221226

"Recent studies have indicated the significance of zinc in neurodegeneration after transient global ischemia. After ischemia, excess glutamate and zinc, which are released in the synaptic clefts, cause the apoptotic death of the target neurons, and finally lead the pathogenesis of vascular type of dementia."

According to:
5. Serum Iron, Zinc, and Copper Levels in Patients with Alzheimer's Disease: A Replication Study and Meta-Analyses. Wang ZX, Tan L, Wang HF, et al. J Alzheimers Dis. 2015;47(3):565-81. PMID: 26401693 DOI: 10.3233/JAD-143108

"To evaluate whether iron, zinc, and copper levels in serum are disarranged in Alzheimer's disease (AD), we performed meta-analyses of all studies on the topic published from 1984 to 2014 and contextually carried out a replication study in serum as well."

"Our meta-analysis results showed that serum zinc was significantly lower in AD patients. Our replication and meta-analysis results showed that serum copper was significantly higher in AD patients than in healthy controls, so our findings were consistent with the conclusions of four previously published copper meta-analyses."

About the Author:

Allen Huff is a principal owner of Precisions Spinal Car and has been a Doctor of Chiropractic for sixteen years. He has a Bachelor's Degree in Biology, worked in student science labs for three years and then obtained his Doctor of Chiropractic from Palmer in 2000. He is passionate about science and is a life-long learner. Allen has a deep desire to use his skills and his knowledge to put the puzzle pieces of his research together in an easy-to-understand format so that he can help people live a healthy life through simple, available, and affordable options.

Allen pursues knowledge through medical journals and then enjoys transcribing the basics of those articles in such a way that people can have access to the information hidden away there. Not many people read those journals, nor have they read the breadth of material that Allen devours. Allen consolidates this data and wants to share his findings with the many persons suffering from cancer. It is his hope that people will feel empowered, rather than helpless, when they realize these are affordable, simple and available options for them to help themselves fight this disease. Best of all, he is not selling any products beyond this e-book. May it bring health and hope to all who read it.

When he is not reading, working in the clinic, writing, you will find Allen enjoying his family at home, being involved attending his daughter's activities, or church functions.

To my readers: Should you discover anything in research that is helpful, an error in the book, or find something you consider needs to be in the next version, please email me book@nucca.info. If I use it, I'll put a thank you to you in the next addition and provide you the next version. Please put the title of the book in the subject line.

Please help me get the word out by writing a review, letting your friends know on Twitter & Facebook. Perhaps suggest it to your friends for a quick book of the month study.

Acknowledgement to the public from Allen: as I have a passion for science and math, I ask for forgiveness of any English or grammatical errors below. The goal of the work is to bring out the facts in a simple, digestible manner but if I used a semicolon vs. a comma or have tenses wrong, please accept my apologies ahead.

Definitions:

The odds ratio (OR) is the proportion of subjects in the treatment group with an outcome divided by the proportion of subjects in a comparison group with the outcome.

The relative risk or "risk ratio" (RR) is the probability of an outcome occurring in a treatment group divided by the probability of an outcome occurring in a comparison group.

A RR or OR of 1 indicates no difference between the treatment and comparison groups. Values greater than 1 favor the treatment group, while values less than 1 favor the comparison group.

The number needed to treat (NNT) provides the number of patients who need to be treated before seeing one patient improve who would not have improved without the intervention. The NNT can infer clinical effectiveness: a high NNT indicates a less effective treatment, and may render the intervention prohibitive. For more information on the NNT and how to calculate it, the reader is referred to: http://en.wikipedia.org/wiki/Number_needed_to_treat

One of the most meaningful, yet misunderstood and underutilized statistics in interpreting clinical research may be the confidence interval (CI). The CI is the certainty that a range (interval) of values contains the true, accurate value of a population that would be obtained if the experiment were repeated. Fortunately, more researchers and reviewers are using CIs to report results of clinical trials in the literature; however, clinicians need to understand the clinical interpretation and value of reporting the CI.

CIs are reported with a "point estimate" (PE) from the sample tested from the population. The PE is a specific value (which may be a sample mean, difference score, effect size, etc), but does NOT represent a "true" value; rather, it represents the "best estimate" of the true value from the average of the sample

The hazard ratio (HR) is the ratio of the hazard rates corresponding to the conditions described by two levels of an explanatory variable. For example, in a drug study, the treated population may die at twice the rate per unit time as the control population. The hazard ratio would be 2, indicating higher hazard of death from the treatment. Or in another study, men receiving the same treatment may suffer a certain complication ten times more frequently per unit time than women, giving a hazard ratio of 10.